Appetites and identities

Appetites and Identities is a clear, inviting and fascinating introduction to the social anthropology of western Europe. It covers
food, migration, politics, urban and country life, magic, religion,
sex and language in an accessible and straightforward fashion,
introducing the student to aspects of the anthropology of contemporary European culture from mussel farmers in the Netherlands
to Basque chambermaids in Lourdes, and from unhappy bachelors
in western Ireland to unwitchers in Portugal. Its scope takes in
Turkey, Greece and Cyprus in the east, to the fringes of Wales,
Scotland and Ireland in the west.

Avoiding the technical language of many anthropological textbooks, *Appetites and Identities* sets out the anthropological literature
on the rich diversity of dialects, cultures and everyday lives of
western European people, offering fascinating insights into how
each region and community differs from its counterparts, despite
the notion of an integrated Europe. The book will stimulate curiosity about social anthropological investigation, and about life in
Europe today.

Students of European Studies, European Languages, EEC
Studies and Sociology, as well as students beginning anthropology
courses and their lecturers, will find this book useful.

Sara Delamont is the Reader in Sociology at the University of
Wales, Cardiff. Her previous books include *Knowledgeable Women*
and *Fieldwork in Educational Settings*.

Appetites and identities

An introduction to the social anthropology of western Europe

Sara Delamont

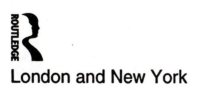

London and New York

First published 1995
by Routledge
11 New Fetter Lane, London EC4P 4EE

Simultaneously published in the USA and Canada
by Routledge
29 West 35th Street, New York, NY 10001

Typeset in Baskerville by LaserScript, Mitcham, Surrey
Printed and bound in Great Britain by
Biddles Ltd, Guildford and King's Lynn

British Library Cataloguing in Publication Data
A catalogue record for this book is available from the British
Library.

Library of Congress Cataloging in Publication Data
Delamont, Sara, 1947–
    Appetites and identities: an introduction to the social
    anthropology of western Europe/Sara Delamont.
    p. cm.
    Includes bibliographical references and index.
    1. Ethnology – Europe. 2. Europe – Social life and customs.
    I. Title.
    D1056.D45   1994
    306.4′094 – dc20   94-9581
                                                       CIP

ISBN 0–415–06253–5 (hbk)
ISBN 0–415–06254–3 (pbk)

Contents

Illustrations

Preface

This is a book about the diverse cultures which exist in western Europe, drawn from the research done by social anthropologists, written for non-anthropologists, indeed for the non-social scientist. It is designed for students studying European languages and cultures, doing degrees in European studies, plus those taking courses in the sociology, politics or anthropology of Europe. The perspective is anthropological, but the book is written for people who have *no* prior knowledge of social anthropology.

All the chapters have titles taken from the poems of J. Elroy Flecker (1947), who died, aged only 31, in 1915. He wrote lovingly of both the northern and the Mediterranean regions of Europe.

A CAVEAT FOR ANTHROPOLOGISTS

This book over-simplifies anthropology and presents a rather static and old-fashioned picture of the discipline. I read social anthropology, and have recently been doing research on social anthropologists, so I know that the way the discipline is presented here will be resented by scholars in that tradition. I have done this deliberately, cold-bloodedly, and ruthlessly. For fifteen years I have been teaching anthropological materials to modern language students who have no social science training, and have discovered that they find the books and journals of social anthropology mystifying. They are perplexed by material I set them to read, repulsed by the technical vocabulary and the theoretical assumptions, puzzled by the data collection methods and convinced that their personal experiences in Spain or Italy are more 'up to date'. This book is for them.

If anthropologists find it useful – either in its own terms or as a shining example of how the discipline can be betrayed by an ignorant outsider – that is a bonus.

Acknowledgements

I have been lucky enough to teach a course on the Mediterranean area to undergraduates studying for the degree scheme in European Community Studies at the University of Wales College of Cardiff since 1978. The students who have taken my course have taught me a great deal in that time. In particular Suzanne Fletcher, Reuben Gates, David Westwood and Claire Turnbull deserve my thanks. I have also learned a great deal about the topics covered in this book from Chris Bettinson, Margaret Kenna, Paul Littlewood, Ralph Grillo, Mike Herzfeld, Costas Adoniou, Mary Darmanin and Zak Palios.

Pat Harris, Elizabeth Renton, Sharen Bechares and Janet Stephens wordprocessed this manuscript for me, and Anna Weaver also checked the bibliography, a really grotty task. I am grateful to all five of them, but particularly to Janet.

This book is dedicated to the memory of Sir Edmund Leach who taught me to love anthropology, and to Paul Atkinson who taught me to love Greece.

Chapter 1

Travellers on a hill
Introduction to the social anthropology of western Europe

like two travellers on a hill, who stay
Viewing the smoke that dims the busy plains . . .

(Flecker, 1947: 49)

INTRODUCTION

The book is intended for two audiences. First there are people
studying 'European Societies', or 'European Community Studies',
or some sub-set of the countries in Europe, who are not anthropologists. This group – including, for example, a British student of
Cypriot origin doing a degree in Greek and French – is my main
target audience. Secondly, there are sociology, geography or
anthropology students who need an introductory overview of the
anthropology of western Europe.

It is called *Appetites and Identities* because it celebrates the variety
of tastes (in food, drink, family life, language and religion) and the
variety of identities that can be found in western Europe.

This is a book about the lives of ordinary people in western
Europe, and celebrates the diversity of life. It is intended for people
doing a wide range of courses, and the idea is that the findings of
anthropology throw light on many aspects of life in western Europe
which remain puzzling without them. Thus the volume starts with
food: the source of much tension, dispute and mutual mis-
understanding in contemporary Europe. Then there are chapters on
farming and fishing; on refugees, migrants and tourists; on peripheral regions; on cities; on local politics; on religion; on gender and
on language. The reader who works through the book will understand the western European diversity and similarity much better, and
have absorbed some social anthropology.

Because there will be readers unfamiliar with social anthropology there is a glossary of some anthropological terms at the end of the book and a list of the places mentioned in the text where research has been conducted, with a reference to a publication on it. Most of the place names are *pseudonyms* to protect the real people who live in that village or neighbourhood.

There is now a large literature on the social anthropology of western Europe with far too many books and articles to include in detail in one volume. To cut down the material, this text *only* deals with research published in English, which means that scholars who are British and American, or those from other countries who publish in English, are the dominant voices. A few French scholars, whose work has been translated and published in English, are the only representatives of other anthropological traditions. The 'Babel tongues' of Chapter 10 are the many languages of the peoples studied by anthropologists, not the languages of the books and articles synthesised.

A second strategy for dealing with the large literature also serves to differentiate this book from Davis (1977), a classic introduction to the social anthropology of the Mediterranean area. I have tried to draw my examples from monographs and journal articles which are not well known, or have been published since Davis wrote, so that this book reads very differently from Davis (1977). Each chapter includes a few case studies where detailed ethnographic material is available, chosen to illustrate the points made. At the end of each chapter is an activity and/or a particular text suggested for further reading which will introduce the reader to the style of anthropological research and to its literature and/or its understandings.

This chapter introduces five key issues which have to be grasped before the rest of the volume makes sense. These include the concept of cultural relativism, the research methods used by anthropologists, 'going native', the history of anthropological research in Europe and its difficulties, and a note on the geographical scope of the book. Before these major themes, there is a caveat for anthropologists. This book simplifies the anthropology of Europe, in that it leaves out some of the most theoretically stretching debates, and some of the fascinating details (such as Ott's 1981 material on 'blessed bread') and treats the texts of anthropologists in an unproblematic way. A course for anthropology students would necessarily have to encompass the theories important in the subject, face the complexities of stories such as

Ott's, and treat the texts as socially constructed (Atkinson, 1990, 1992). Students studying 'French Language and Society' courses neither need nor want, nor have the social science background, to follow such debates, which are simply ignored in this volume.

The main purpose of the book is to show that western Europe contains many diverse cultures, which are not simply bounded by nation states. There are communities which have existed much longer than the nation states which now encompass them, and cultures which cross national boundaries. To understand the present it may be necessary to look back a thousand years, or examine geographical similarities across borders. Thus the modern inhabitant of the Friuli area of Italy (Holmes, 1989) has similarities with the heretics persecuted there in the sixteenth and seventeenth centuries (Ginzburg, 1980, 1983). Hostilities between Serbs and Croats have *some* roots in the separation of the Catholic and Orthodox Christian churches and the sacking of Constantinople by Crusaders in 1204. Modern nation states, and multinational organisations cannot wipe away these continuities. Equally, national boundaries may divide people whose way of life is very similar. The everyday life of a woman in a French Alpine village is more similar to that of her equivalent in an Italian, Swiss or Austrian Alpine village than it is to an urban Frenchwoman, or a village woman in Brittany or Lorraine, or on the Languedoc coast, yet she *is* still 'French', not Italian, Swiss or Austrian.

Anthropologists have studied a range of diverse lifestyles all over Europe, and this book is a celebration of the multiple cultures and multiple populations of western Europe.

A book can only synthesise material which exists. Most of the material discussed in this volume is on Eire, the UK, Portugal, Spain, some regions of France (especially Brittany), Italy, Greece, Cyprus, Malta and The Netherlands. Germany, Austria and Belgium, are mentioned occasionally, while Denmark, Norway, Sweden, Finland and Luxembourg are largely absent, because there are relatively few studies by social anthropologists available in English. When the chapters are focused on immigration, or guestworkers or refugees, residents of western Europe whose origins are in Turkey or Serbia or Tunisia or other labour-exporting countries are mentioned briefly. This reflects the published work by anthropologists in English *not* the political importance of the countries, or the density of their populations, or the power of their economies. The themes chosen for the book are equally relevant to all countries, but the illustrative material is not equally available.

CULTURAL RELATIVISM

Cultural relativism is a grand-sounding phrase, but it is an essential part of how anthropological researchers collect their data, and not difficult to understand. When we come across something that is done a different way from the one we are used to, it is easy to judge it as 'wrong' (or peculiar, or revolting, or immoral, or unnatural). If you have always slept at night and been up during the day, it would seem odd to move to a culture where people were nocturnal. If you have grown up wearing clothes, a nudist colony would be embarrassing, and might seem immoral. Food is an area where it is hard to accept other people's way of doing things. If you grew up in a traditional Yorkshire home, where the Yorkshire pudding was served with gravy as a separate course before the roast beef and vegetables, then you would find it odd to have them served together all on one plate. If you had grown up with them served together, getting a plate of Yorkshire pudding and gravy on their own would seem odd. Being a good researcher involves suspending judgement, and focusing on why people do what they do, believe what they believe, eat what they eat, drink what they drink and say what they say, in their culture. A good example of a researcher putting his own ideas aside so he could understand another culture is Crapanzano's (1985) book on Afrikaners in South Africa. He hated everything they stood for, but put that aside to study how they saw their world. Researchers in Europe are not likely to come across practices and beliefs as far from their own as anthropologists who study Indians in the South American rainforest or the aboriginal inhabitants of the Malay peninsula, but cultural relativism is still needed. A simple example will suffice.

Patrick Leigh Fermor and a companion were in a small town on the coast of mainland Greece called Astakos. It was extremely hot and the taverna had only egg and chips to eat.

> Even at nine in the evening the town was hardly cooler than at noon . . . It had been a day of heat, glare, loss, breakdown and illness . . . After half an hour the old woman clip-clopped out of the shadows with a plate in either hand. 'I'm sorry they've been so long', she said kindly. 'It's the cooling that eats up the time.'

'The cooling?'

'Hot food is bad. It makes people ill.'

I remembered that this belief prevails in certain remote regions. Hot fried eggs are especially dangerous and a prudent cook sets them aside until they seize up. The yolks stiffen to discs of yellow cardboard in a matrix of white glâcé kid islanded in cold oil . . .

(1966: 149)

Fermor and his companion could not face eating these eggs, and most readers of this book probably could not eat them either. However, as a proper researcher it is advisable not only to eat them, but to accept while 'in the field' the belief that hot food is bad for humans, and to include the set of ideas about hot and cold and healthy and unhealthy foods in the research. Failure to adapt to such beliefs will not only impede the research, in that the locals will be constantly reminded that the researcher is *not* a local, it will also close off an avenue for exploring the culture you have come to study. In August 1992 the British weekly magazine *Women's Own* published the results of a survey of 1,000 women, done by a leading market research firm, on their knowledge of the EEC. The results showed that British women were very ignorant about the EEC. Only 69 per cent of the women knew that Britain was a member of the EEC, and 92 per cent could not list the twelve members; 40 per cent did not know who Jacques Delors was, replying that he was a racing driver, a fashion designer or a kind of perfume; only 30 per cent knew what the EEC was, and half did not know what Maastricht was including one person who thought it was a Dutch cheese.

Given this level of ignorance, prejudices can flourish completely unchecked. However, prejudices are not dispelled by knowledge alone. Knowing Denmark is a member of the EEC does not dispel prejudices against Danes, or the Danish government fishing policy, or make British pig farmers think more kindly of the Danish bacon marketing policies. However, if one can cultivate an attitude of cultural relativism, it is possible to understand why Danish fishing policy takes the form it does. At a local level, if you found yourself in the Dutch village of St Gerlach on the second Saturday in June you might wonder why there was an enormous traffic jam, but if you read Bax (1985b) you would know the cars were being blessed by the local monks in the name of St Gerlach, and you would understand why. Even if you were not interested in having the monks bless *your* car, you could be sympathetic to the motives of these clogging up the streets. Similarly once you have read Campbell (1964), Machin (1983) or Stewart (1991), and discovered that phantoms (*fantakta*) appear at mid-day in rural Greece, you would appreciate why country-dwellers are so committed to a siesta that keeps respectable people in their homes.

There is a danger as severe as failing to adopt cultural relativity: that is 'going native', discussed after the methods used by social anthropologists have been explained.

HOW ARE DATA COLLECTED?

To understand the material used in this book it is useful to know how the data are collected. There are two ways to find out what social anthropologists do: textbooks on methods and auto-biographical accounts by researchers of what they did. Textbooks on methods usually set out what researchers ought to do, while scholars' autobiographies usually tell stories about how everything *nearly* went wrong and the research *nearly* failed altogether. A good textbook on how to do the sort of research described in this book is Hammersley and Atkinson (1983), and the book by Pina-Cabral and Campbell (1992) is a collection of autobiographical accounts. Most of the books mentioned in this volume have some account of how the data were collected, often tucked away in an appendix, but sometimes early on, like Barrett (1974: 4–22). Because this is a book written for people who are strangers to anthropology, I have described an imaginary piece of research, to illustrate what anthropologists do. The main methods used are briefly described, but not all researchers would be comfortable with all of them, not all 'work' in every setting, not all are possible for every scholar, and not everyone is interested in the data they generate. After the imaginary project invented to display possible ways a scholar can get data, some examples of actual autobiographical material from anthropologists are given.

Central to anthropology is *fieldwork*. This does not mean working in a field, but choosing a place to stay and going to live in it, which is known as being 'in the field'. A typical anthropologist is about 22 or 23 when she starts her first, and most important piece of research, her first proper fieldwork. The account of 'Rachel Verinder's' fieldwork is based on autobiographical accounts published by successful anthropologists and interviews with twenty-four social anthropology PhD students in Britain done during 1991 as part of a research project.

Imagine Rachel Verinder has graduated in social anthropology, and has been offered a scholarship to do a PhD at Boarbridge University. She and her thesis supervisor, Dr Selina Goby, decide that Rachel should do research on Galicians and the Galician regionalist and separatist movement (Galicia is a region in north-western Spain). Rachel did 'A' level Spanish and has spent several holidays there since, and she is interested in Atlantic maritime cultures, the lives of women in fishing communities and regionalist movements in Europe. For nine months Rachel stays in Boarbridge, improving her knowledge of social anthropology, especially the anthropology of Europe and of maritime societies, reading about Galicia, and other regions of Spain, and learning the Galician dialect/language. Then she packs appropriate clothes and equipment for collecting data, such as a camera, tape-recorder and lots of notebooks and pens, and sets off from Boarbridge for the ferry to Santander. When she lands in Spain she heads for Galicia, and searches out a fishing village where she will live for the next year or more. She has to try several villages before she finds one that has a bus service to the nearest town, has a family who are prepared to rent her a room, and has fishing boats still working.

Once settled, Rachel is 'in the field', and she can start her fieldwork. The most important part is living in the village, and watching what goes on. Where feasible Rachel will do things with people in the village, where it is not feasible to join in, she will watch what she is allowed to. Once the villagers have got used to her being around, watching is supplemented with talking. Rachel talks informally to everyone possible, does formal interviews with people, collecting their family trees and hearing their life stories, plus gathering folk tales and songs, listening to gossip, jokes and legends.

A fieldworker is likely to draw maps of the village, of the insides of houses, of the graveyard, diagrams of the seating plans at weddings or funerals, the layout of fishing boats and anything else which has a spatial angle. Rachel will count the number of residents in the village, count the fishing boats, measure the sizes of fields, orchards and pastures, count cows, sheep and pigs, estimate the size of the fishing catch, work out how many tourists come, how many people get the bus each day, how many cars, taxis, motor scooters and even bicycles there are, how many pupils in the school and so on. It will be important to hear who speaks Galician and who does not, and when Galician and Castilian (Spanish) are used. If Rachel is allowed on a fishing boat she will go, if not she will find out why women are not allowed to sail on them. The lives of the women will probably be easier for her to observe than those of men. If there is separatist political activity, Rachel will try to attend any meetings, meet the activists and discover what is motivating them.

Apart from what she can see, and what she can learn by listening and asking, there may also be documents. Rachel might spend days in the provincial capital working on municipal archival material, or in the cathedral or ecclesiastical records, or both. If the Galician regionalist movement has produced newsletters, or pamphlets, or books, these will all be read. Rachel might get the schoolchildren to write her something, or ask to read letters sent home by villagers living abroad.

As Rachel goes on living in the village she will find that she has been told different things by different people and she will set out to find out why. As her Galician improves, she will spot that people were lying to her, and find out why they did so. (It is common, for example, for villagers to think that outsiders are tax inspectors, CIA agents, spies or other undesirables.) As her understanding of the people and the place deepens, Rachel will be able to come up with more and more questions to ask: to cross-check her ideas, to corroborate earlier information, to test her developing hypotheses. She also makes friends and gets involved.

At the end of her year or more, Rachel packs up her stuff and returns to Boarbridge. There she sorts out her data and picks a central theme with which to organise them. Using anthropological theory, and organising her data around that theme she writes a PhD thesis. Once that is done, she starts to publish articles about 'her' village, and to write a book. That takes a considerable time, so that if Rachel spent 1993 in her village, the book would probably appear in 1997 or so. Jane Cowan, for example, did her main fieldwork in Sohos in the 1983–85 period, got her PhD in 1988, and published her book in 1990 (a speedy publication). If we imagine Rachel's career after her PhD, she would hope to get a lectureship and to return to Galicia periodically over the next ten years or so. She might do her next piece of research on Galicians in some other region of Spain (e.g. Catalonia) or working in another country such as Switzerland (Buechler and Buechler, 1981; Buechler, 1987). She might study another separatist movement, or another fishing area, depending what she was interested in and could get a grant for. By the time she is 35 she would have published her book on her village, and a series of articles on both her first, and her subsequent fieldwork.

Rachel is an imaginary character. However, I invented the story after reading many autobiographical accounts by anthropologists who have studied European countries and after doing a piece of research on twenty-four current doctoral candidates in British anthropology. Some people go alone, when they are as young as 'Rachel'. Other anthropologists are older and some do their field research with their spouse and sometimes also their children. For example, Scheper-Hughes (1979: 9) went to live in Ballybran, on the west coast of Ireland, with her husband and three children:

> The research team was the family – myself, my husband, and our three children: Jenny, aged five, Sarah, aged two, and Nathanael, five months at the start of fieldwork. We could hardly avoid being *participant* observers in the community as we shared with the hardy villagers day in and day out their life style, their celebrations, their ennui and depressions, during the seemingly endless winter, their fear of the truly awesome wind storms that rocked the peninsula, and their joy at the coming of spring – the flowing of cow's milk and the birth of the calves and lambs. We worshipped with them on Sundays and holy days; we confessed our sins to the same curate, we visited their old and sick, and mourned with them their dead.

The children were part of the research.

> My elder daughter attended the local primary school, where she learned bilingual reading, math, her prayers, sewing, Irish dancing and music and how to duck the bamboo rod.

Scheper-Hughes's husband became a teacher at the local secondary school, and was also able to spend time in the all-male pub.

Similarly, Galt (1991) went into the field in southern Italy with his wife and 7-year-old son; Sydel Silverman (1975) went to Montecastello di Vibio with her husband and had a baby while in the town. Some couples have done fieldwork together and both published their findings, such as John and Maria Corbin (1983), John Hutson (1971) and Susan Hutson (1971), and George and Louise Spindler (1987).

The age, marital status and lifestyle of the anthropologists will have an impact on the people they are studying, and sensitive researchers use this as a data collection stragegy and build it into their reports and analysis.

Researchers who go into the field alone like Rachel may be seen as rather unusual by the community they choose. Rosenberg (1988: xiii) went to her French Alpine village alone, and the inhabitants were puzzled: 'over what a young girl was doing alone in their village. Eventually, someone took me aside and asked me if my mother knew where I was.' Similarly, Cowan (1990: 54): 'As a young, foreign, solitary woman coming to stay in a town where I had neither relatives nor even compatriots, I must have seemed to most Sohoians tremendously out of place.'

Single men can also be seen as odd. Chapman (1992: 42–43) studied a rural community in Brittany:

> If you come into rural Brittany, as a young and educated person, there are two quite different local models of your status, more or less morally polarised: either you are a long-haired work-shy drop-out, failing in all the essential local virtues like getting on and working hard (why else, otherwise, would a good education have landed you in a dump like Plouturiec?), or you are an aspiring young professional, whose visit to Brittany is part of a career structure.

Chapman learnt that the second role was preferable, and his 'well-meaning' friends in Brittany imposed this role on him. He was a scholar from Oxford whose career *necessitated* time in Plouturiec, just as a young doctor might have to spend some time in a rural area.

The motives of anthropologists are often mystifying to the people they have come to study, and they may be accused of espionage or worse. For example when Belmonte (1989: 11) was trying to get established in a poor neighbourhood of Naples, he met resistance.

> Although I succeeded in making friends with three young working men and became quite a celebrity at their nightly hangout, I attracted the attention of other people in the neighbourhood who decided my anthropologist pose was a clever disguise. I had to be a police agent or a spy of some sort. There was enough illegal activity going on to make people afraid of me. My new friends

were criticized for associating with me, and I was threatened with a beating if I persisted in my attempt to live in the area.

Aschenbrenner (1986: viii) was first in Karpofora only two years after the military coup of 1967.

> Initially, villagers had some problem with the reason I declared for wanting to be in their midst, namely, to learn the language and then their customs and the history of the village . . . they doubted that these were my real reasons . . . As I learned after a couple of years, people very commonly believed that the CIA of the United States was not only deeply involved in the 1967 *coup d'état* but was also active in the current affairs of Greece. Hence it was expectable that in 1969 villagers had an initial inclination to wonder if I were a CIA agent.

Aschenbrenner therefore carefully avoided studying anything to do with contemporary politics.

When O'Neill (1987: 17) arrived on the bus at Fontelas, on the border between northern Portugal and Galicia, two cows had just been stolen, and the villagers were sure they had been taken over the border by Galicians. O'Neill spoke Galician, and: 'I was thus suspected not merely of being a suspicious student, a government spy, a land surveyor, a professional contrabandist, but also a cattle thief.'

Luckily the cattle were found in Galicia and O'Neill was able to convince the villagers that he was not the thief.

Whether alone or in a family, the researcher chooses a community, finds a house or flat or room to rent, and starts trying to gather data. It is usual to concentrate on one or more aspects of life in the culture being studied, but equally, usual not to finalise what these aspects will be until some time in the setting has elapsed.

For example, among the recent Greek projects Cowan (1990) is a study of dance and of gender; Stewart (1991) of masculinity, shepherding and beliefs in the supernatural; Herzfeld (1991) of the impact of conservation ideology on the Cretan town of Rethemnos; Seremetakis (1991) is about death and divination in the Mani; Danforth (1989) about fire walking; and Hirschon (1989) a refugee community's separate identity fifty years after its arrival in Athens in 1922.

Researchers discover that a particular feature of 'their' village or neighbourhood is particularly important to its inhabitants; or has not been studied properly before; or is something happening while they are in the field (an election, a new road, a tourist development, a rare festival); or that they are able to get good data on some features of the place and not on others. The scholar may also be impelled by a theoretical debate, or by a conviction that previous researchers were wrong about the culture, or by access to new kind of data. Choices about the focus of research are not taken lightly, and the strength of anthropology lies in its ability to focus on what members of a culture value or think important, rather than what the researcher thinks important before entering the field.

The types of data that a researcher can collect will also be limited by their age, sex, marital status and race. Aschenbrenner went to Karpofora in 1969:

> as a 40-year-old single male. In accordance with the villagers' sense of propriety this meant that I was 'naturally' most often in the company of males, usually adults. Thus my exposure to women, youth and children has been more limited, tending quite often to be only when one or more village males were present.
>
> (1986: vii)

Campbell (1992: 153) writes similarly, and this theme is further discussed in Chapter 9.

Learning the language is an important part of anthropological fieldwork. Fears that one's grasp of the language is inadequate compound the apprehension that always accompanies the start of fieldwork. Take Belmonte (1989: 1):

> I arrived in Naples on a cold, wet, abysmally gray day of early April. I was frightened and apprehensive. I didn't speak more than a few sentences of Italian, and I was geographically lost.

Mastering the language is often the researcher's first task. So when Aschenbrenner (1986) studied Karpofora from 1969 onwards he began by concentrating on his Greek because: 'I felt a persistent anxiety about my command of Modern Greek that drove me to devote several hours daily to language study' (p. vi).

One reason that anthropologists interested in southern Italy distrust the book by Banfield (1958) is that he did not speak Italian or the dialect of Calabrian used in Montegrano. Many field sites are in places where dialects are spoken; or where minority languages like Provençal or Basque are an important symbol of identity; or where language is a political issue. In Ballybran, for

example, Irish Gaelic was symbolically and even financially important (it attracted government grants) (Scheper-Hughes, 1979).
Older and wealthier researchers may hire an assistant/interpreter
to help. Galt (1991) employed 'a field assistant – really colleague –
named Giorgio Cardone who helped with arranging and carrying
out formal interviews . . . inculcating in me a smattering of the
local dialect . . .'. Galt already had Italian, but not the dialect of the
heel of Italy. Anthropologists routinely need to spend time learning a language before they start fieldwork, then find it is necessary
to improve their linguistic skills to do fieldwork properly, and
often discover that language, accent and dialect are important in
their field site. That is the focus of Chapter 10.

Not all fieldwork is successful. There are people who die in the
field, those who find that they are unable to gather decent data,
and those who never write up what they did collect. The studies
used in this book all 'made it' at least as far as being PhD theses,
and most of them became journal articles or books. The next
section focuses on one particularly insidious form of failure, which
the researchers may not even recognise themselves.

'GOING NATIVE'

Going native is an objectionable term, deservedly, for an objectionable phenomenon. It means over-identifying with the respondents, and losing the researcher's twin perspectives of her own
culture and, more importantly, of her 'research' outlook. Many
classic anthropological jokes or folk tales turn on 'going native':
stories of reaching the sacred burial ground of a tribe to find a
ceremony in progress, only to discover that the leading ritual
expert is another anthropologist, whipping lazy locals into the
correct form of the dances. Students are warned of the last great
Kwakiutl potlatch: attended by ten bored Kwakiutl and twenty
eager anthropologists.

Anthropologists have particular problems trying to handle this.
Loring Danforth (1989) highlights the problem of 'contemporary
anthropology in a post-modern world'. He describes how he began
his Greek research (on death rituals and fire walking).

I was an American, a graduate student in anthropology, and I
had been brought up as a member of a liberal Protestant church
in a white, upper-middle-class suburb of Boston. I was going to

live in a Greek village, a warm emotional place where people ate exotic food outdoors late at night and men embraced each other in public . . . Greek churches were filled with candles, bearded priests dressed in splendid robes.

(1989: 189)

Danforth was obviously in danger of falling in love with Greece. The danger is always a real one. If our heroine, Rachel Verinder, is going to be a successful researcher, she has to go to her Galician fishing village and come home again to Boarbridge with her data. She is a failure if she hates the staple diet so much she comes home after a week, saying the villagers are barbarians. However, she is also a failure if she becomes more Galician than the Galicians. If Rachel stops writing her diary, collecting and recording data, and thinking like an anthropologist, and becomes a leading light of the Galician separatist movement, then she has 'gone native'. Suppose Dr Selina Goby comes to visit Rachel and finds Rachel leading the protest march on Madrid, or planting a bomb in the police post, or organising a school boycott; then Dr Goby would have every reason to accuse Rachel of 'going native'.

Every anthropology department has a story about a promising student who set out to do a study of Italian circus performers or French gypsies or Belgian waffle makers and never came back. He or she can be seen walking the highwire in Naples, or begging in Avignon, or selling waffles in Bruges, lost to scholarship.

Even among those who come home, and produce books and articles, there may be cases of 'over-rapport' or 'going native'. It is arguable, for example, that Herzfeld, whose many publications on Greece will be cited in this book, is so enamoured of Greece that he has lost his scholarly detachment. Some of the books produced on Europe give a sense of researchers who fell in love with the culture they had come to study and lost their critical faculties. Gilmore (1980), for example, accuses many of the researchers who had studied Andalusia before him of 'going native' among the middle and upper classes, so that they failed to appreciate how grim life is among the poorest, landless day-labourers. Some male researchers may be blind to the harshness of women's existence, some female researchers may be too entangled in women's lives to recognise men's realities, and so on. When you go on, as I hope you will, to read the best of the books published by the anthropologists studying Europe, you will want to be alert to spot those who over-identify with 'their' fieldwork site.

The final theme of this chapter is the development of the European research done by anthropologists and its strengths and weaknesses.

THE DEVELOPMENT OF THE RESEARCH

Most of the authors who have reviewed the anthropology of the Mediterranean area, or of Europe, date their specialism from the publication of Julian Pitt-Rivers's (1954) *The People of the Sierra* (see, for example, Boissevain, 1977). Pitt-Rivers was an upper-class Englishman who went to live in a tiny village in Andalusia, Spain, in 1948. Franco was in charge of a police state, a dictatorship; the legacy of the Spanish Civil War was continuing bitterness between winners and losers. In the 1950s two researchers, John Campbell, a British war veteran, and Ernestine Friedl an American, began research in Greece, leading to Campbell (1964) and Friedl (1962). However, long before Pitt-Rivers, in the 1930s, a woman from Chicago called Charlotte Gower Chapman had done an ethnography of a Sicilian community (Milocca) although it lay as an unpublished (and unknown) doctoral thesis until 1971. Pitkin (1985) first went to Italy in 1951 and Wylie (1957) conducted his research on Peyrane – a village in southern France – in 1950/51.

These studies of Mediterranean life were the parallels of a set of projects done in the Celtic fringe of Europe. A classic study of farming families in County Clare, Ireland had been published in 1940 by Arensberg and Kimball, two Americans. This was followed by studies in Wales (Rees, 1950; Frankenberg, 1957; Rees and Davies, 1960; Emmett, 1964), Scotland (Littlejohn, 1964) and a marginal agricultural area of England (Williams, 1956).

The northern European countries were also being studied from the 1950s onwards. Turney-High (1953) began studying Château-Gérard (Belgium) in 1949, while Spindler (1973) studied a German village, Burgbach, from 1960 onwards.

The search for origins – for the 'real' beginning of the anthropology of Europe is not the purpose of this book, although the interested reader can consult Boissevain (1975, 1977, 1979), Cole (1977), Crump (1975), Davis (1977), Fernandez (1987), Freeman (1973), Gilmore (1990), Herzfeld (1987), Llobera (1986), Pina-Cabral (1992).

These are all reviews of the research, and all discuss whether there is a meaningful category of 'Mediterranean anthropology' or 'anthropology of Europe'; and if so, whose work 'belongs' to the various traditions. There is no need for a beginner to become embroiled in such disputes, and none is dealt with here. For this chapter, only one feature of the research is important: its lopsidedness.

Most of the population of Europe lives in cities or towns, and most people do not grow their own grain for flour, rear their own animals for meat, milk their own cow or sheep, catch their own fish, harvest their own grapes for their own wine, or pick their own oranges from the trees. The people studied by anthropologists have mostly been those who *do* do these things, living in rural areas and engaging in subsistence production. For every study of factory workers or bus drivers or bank clerks or shop owners or tour guides there are ten or twenty studies of rural communities in that country. Davis (1977) was scathing about this bias when describing Mediterranean anthropology:

> The desire to be as primitive as every other colleague may be equally responsible for two other failures which must be mentioned here. Mediterraneanists have chosen to work in the marginal areas of the region – in the mountains, in the small peasant communities, in the tribal hinterlands of the Maghreb.
>
> (Davis, 1977: 7)

It is not only the researchers on the Mediterranean who work in the marginal areas. There are more studies of Scottish crofting than of Glasgow; more of Welsh villages than of Cardiff; more of rural Brittany than of Rennes and Nantes and so on. As Davis said (1977: 7):

> Anthropology is only anthropology if it is done very much abroad, in unpleasant conditions, in societies which are very different from the ethnographer's native habitat, very different from the sort of place where he [sic] might go on holiday.

Anthropologists feel happier if their fieldwork site is in a remote place, away from civilisation and comfort. Rosenberg (1988: xi) feels obliged to point out that:

> I loved living in France and was amused when my anthropologist colleagues who worked in more exotic locales asked me about my time in the bush. I would bravely attempt to match

their stories of hardship by pointing out that 'my village' was more than twenty-four hours away from the nearest three-star restaurant.

This is a joke, but like all the best jokes, Rosenberg is making a serious point about anthropology.

THE DIFFICULTIES OF EUROPEAN ANTHROPOLOGY

Apart from impressing *other* anthropologists with the harshness and remoteness of one's field site, there are some genuine problems associated with doing anthropology in cultures which are actually your own, or are close to home. There are several collections of papers in which anthropologists discuss these problems. American anthropologists faced their difficulties in Messerschmidt (1982), and British ones in Jackson (1987). Most recently, Pina-Cabral and Campbell (1992) addresses the same problems.

For the non-anthropologist the problems may seem trivial, and the scholars' discussions self-indulgent. However, it is important to recognise that when studying something that is familiar it is easy to miss important features of the culture precisely because they *are* familiar. For example, when mentioning Scheper-Hughes's work in Ballybran earlier in this chapter I said the bars were male-only territory. Many readers of this book would not find that strange or unlikely: it would only be a 'finding' if the bars had been only for women, or only for people over 60, or only for children under 10. A good researcher needs to make everything problematic, even things which are 'the same' as he or she is used to, and the nearer the culture is to 'home' the harder that is to do.

The other difficulty arises when the researcher falls into the trap of seeing the culture being studied as 'backward', 'primitive' or 'underdeveloped'. This can easily follow from choosing a remote field site, and focusing on the picturesque features of it, forgetting that nowhere in Europe is beyond the reach of mass media and the global economic system. It is salutary to read Susan Rogers's (1991) material on 'her' French villagers in Ste Foy. They thought America was a very backward country due to: 'the relative paucity of services provided or mandated by the American federal government' (p. 195). The French in Ste Foy took for granted: 'national health insurance, paid maternity leave, annual one-month paid vacation' (p. 196) none of which an American has by legal right.

Anyone reading this book needs to recognise that nearly every culture in Europe believes itself to be superior to all others, and that what it eats, drinks, wears, sleeps under and believes in are the 'natural' things all sensible people would choose if they could get them. A unified Europe is only going to work if those who cook in oil can accept that others cook in goose grease and vice versa.

SUGGESTED READING/ACTIVITY

Colin Thubron's (1986) *Journey into Cyprus* is the story of a walk all round the island before the Turkish invasion in 1974 and subsequent partition. This should be available in a public library.

Chapter 2

The golden oranges
Food, appetites and identity

Knowest thou the land where bloom the lemon trees
And darkly gleam the golden oranges?

(Flecker, 1947: 21)

INTRODUCTION

The image of orange and lemon trees is a useful one to start a chapter on food in western Europe. The big division in the EEC is between those who live too far north to see lemon trees in blossom or to pick oranges at the roadside from those for whom citrus fruits are commonplace. The line divides Europe as regards food. North of the line the drink is beer, the food is cooked in animal fat, and there are ample dairy products. South of the line the drink is wine, food is cooked in olive oil, and milk and butter are not central features of the diet.

Compare these two evocations of food.

The cooking of the Mediterranean shores, endowed with all the natural resources, the colour and flavour of the South, is a blend of tradition and brilliant improvisation. The Latin genius flashes from the kitchen pans . . .

The ever recurring elements in the foods throughout these countries are the oil, the saffron, the garlic, the pungent local wines; the aromatic perfume of rosemary, wild marjoram and basil drying in the kitchens; the brilliance of the market stalls piled high with pimentos, aubergines, tomatoes, olives, melons, figs and limes; the great heaps of shiny fish . . . all manner of unfamiliar cheeses from sheep or goat's milk . . .

(David, 1955: 9)

That is the food of the south, now that of the north:

> Fish and freshness, above all salmon, herrings and prawns . . .
> dark, purple-brown reindeer meat . . . smoked pork loin . . .
> close rye bread . . . sweet pale cloudberries . . . sugar and spice
> in unexpected foods . . . aquavit and unfailingly good coffee . . .
> great discs of rye bread, flat and crisp . . . tunbrod, baked
> pancake-thin on a griddle; you cut this into wedges and roll
> them round slices of pickled herring . . . Smoked filleted eels
> . . . tubs of pickled herrings in many varieties . . . black-streaked
> squid, freshwater pollan and pike . . . Another major Scan-
> danavian food . . . is pork . . . The best . . . is the boned, smoked
> loin known as hamburgerryg . . . Wherever you find pork, you
> will find cheese and butter, as pigs are, or were, fed on the skim
> milk and whey . . . The skill of the pastrycooks in Scandanavia
> . . . the fine skill and lightness, the lovely unusual notes of
> aniseed, cardamon and cinnamon . . . the swirls and curls of
> well-buttered dough.
>
> (Grigson, 1983: 160–161)

These are two cookery writers encouraging their readers to enjoy the food of the Mediterranean and of northern Europe. Many elements of the diet are different: olive oil versus butter for frying is only one way in which the cuisines of the south and the north are distinct.

In this chapter the focus is on how food was a crucial element in the origins of the EEC, how tastes differ and why trouble over food is a recurrent feature of life in Brussels and Strasbourg.

There are four themes in the chapter which serve as background to the brief history of the Common Agricultural Policy (CAP) in Chapter 3. The memories of the hunger of the first fifty years of the twentieth century open the chapter. Then there is a section on food as an element in regional, national and local culture, and its symbolic value. This is followed by an equivalent section on drink. Finally there is a section on food preparation as *work*.

Food and drink are central to the EEC. Many of the people running the individual member nations and the EEC organ-isations starved in the 1940s. Dutch, Belgian, German, Greek and French people of 50 or more – the ages of maximum political power – experienced starvation, rationing and food shortages in their own childhood. Anyone over 30 in all European countries had *parents* who lived through poverty and hunger in the 1930s, rationing in the war and shortages in the late 1940s and 1950s.

Only those born in the last twenty years *can* be free of the fear of food shortages. Hunger is the focus of the next section of this chapter. The CAP was designed by people who had starved, and were concerned to stop anyone in the EEC ever starving again.

THE GREAT HUNGER

The UK escaped the starvation of the war and the aftermath. The diet may have been dull, bland and repetitive, but no-one had to eat grass. The continental countries were not so lucky.

Pitkin (1985) is a story of four generations of an Italian family who leave Calabria for Valmonte near Rome in 1933 driven by poverty and hunger, then suffer near starvation during the war and its aftermath, and only get settled with regular food in the 1950s. Similarly, Fraser (1973) is full of memories of elderly Andalusians who were hungry throughout their early lives. Francisco Avila, aged 76, recalls his childhood: 'At least we ate every day and that was saying a lot. We were among the better-off of the poor' (p. 17). His wife, Maria, aged 74, is quoted in more detail about her childhood:

> We all ate out of the same bowl, we didn't have plates. No-one could put their spoon into the bowl until the parents had taken the first dip. In the mornings before work we had coffee. Barley coffee, we couldn't afford the real thing. And with that, if we were lucky, we'd have a sweet potato. If not, nothing. At noon we'd eat soup, with a bit of dried cod in it if it was a good day, a piece of bread and a dried fig.
>
> (p. 21)

After she married Francisco:

> We were able to eat a bit better than most, we had fish more often and every year we killed a pig. From that I cured a couple of legs of *serrano* ham, made sausages, mortadello, black puddings.
>
> (p. 23)

A similar story is told by Pedro Perez, aged 68. He was a day-labourer before the war, which meant being at the vineyard at dawn to start work, a walk of one and a half hours before dawn, on an empty stomach.

We walked to the vineyards on empty stomachs and worked for an hour before a bit of the food we took with us: a pot of bread soup, the sort we make here, a *tortilla*, a few dried figs when we were in luck – that was all we had to eat from dawn until late at night. No-one had more. At noon we had an hour off and ate the rest of our food.

(pp. 28–29)

As Pedro Perez summarized his life at that period: 'I was always hungry – one couldn't get rid of it' (p. 28).

Working-class men were expected to do a full day's work on a diet of the most meagre kind. Shepherds in the French Basque, for example, had a midday meal of 'a thick porridge of ewes' milk and cornmeal bread' (Ott, 1981: 153). In Kippel, a Swiss Alpine village:

During the Depression the potato was the only thing that saved the valley from starvation. One woman recalled that her family was so poor that if they had some cheese to put on their potatoes at dinner they considered themselves fortunate. Bread was out of the question – potatoes and milk kept them alive and healthy . . . No-one died of starvation, and only a few were damaged by malnutrition.

(Friedl, 1974: 30)

Netting (1981) reports the same dependence on the potato in his Swiss village. In northern Spain, in the village studied by Behar (1986: 37): 'The beginnings of this century and especially the period after the Civil War were times of hunger'. Symbols of this hunger in Santa Maria de Monte were barb bread and potato bread. *Pan de picos*, 'barb' bread was made from the seeds of the burdock plant (*cadillo*): 'an older woman remembers children hating it because the burdock barbs inevitably got stuck in the flour'. After the Civil War women put potato into the bread dough: 'Both the "barb bread" and the potato bread were of lower quality than the black rye bread that was the daily fare of most villagers at this time' (p. 37).

These are poor people in peacetime. The Spanish Civil War; the Second World War in France, Germany, the Benelux countries, Greece and Italy; and the Greek civil war, all brought *worse* hunger to the poor – the majority of the population – in all the countries of the European mainland. Even when peace returned, people were poor and their diet was meagre, monotonous and short of animal protein.

When Margaret Kenna (1990) did her first fieldwork on Nisos (a remote Greek island) in 1966/67 the diet of the islanders was simple and largely vegetarian: 'Bean soup, lentil purées and salads of wild greens (*chorta*) made up the major part of the diet for most islanders' (p. 147). Meat was a rare treat: 'Few ate meat regularly, some only three times a year – at Easter, on the Feast of the Assumption in August, and on the feast day of the island's patron saint' (p. 146). If an engagement or wedding came along, or a relative returned from Athens, a meat meal would be provided (chicken, goat or sheep). There were a few rabbits, and some partridge to be hunted, but otherwise sausage and ham from the pig slaughtered in November would be the only meat. Fishing existed, but the majority of farming families could only afford to buy the cheapest species from the fishermen. Fish like sea bream and red mullet, which would have fetched a luxury price in a tourist centre like Rhodes, were unsaleable on Nisos because they were too expensive.

A similar diet is reported from other peasant villages. For example, Moore (1976b: 18) reports that in 1955 the diet of a day-labourer in Los Santos on Tenerife was:

traditional gruel made of wheat and corn flour called *gofio*, fresh vegetables and bananas, occasional fish brought in by some 20 local fishermen from the surrounding low yield waters, and on rare occasions beef, goat or chicken.

The rarity of meat eating partly explains the high prestige attached to the successful sheep thief in Crete (Herzfeld, 1985), Naxos (Stewart, 1991) and Sardinia (Berger, 1986). In all three cultures stealing a sheep from a neighbouring village, cooking and eating it was an accomplishment. In Naxos a skilled thief was a sought-after husband because he was believed to be an audacious and clever man. Stewart (1991: 69) was told a famous Naxiote story in which a 'first-rate thief' was dying, and ordered his two sons to find their sister a husband who was a more skilful thief than they were. The sons' subsequent attempts to outwit the man they chose, who eventually outwits them, turns on stealing and re-stealing a fat lamb. While today Cretan and Naxiote sheep stealing is a contest of symbolic importance, mountain-dwellers told Stewart (1991: 265) that in the past theft was a response to poverty, 'we were hungry and so we stole to eat': taking sheep from richer villages in the lowlands. Berger (1986) in his account of Sardinian shepherds reports similar patterns of animal theft on that island.

Anthropologists working in Europe in the 1970s and 1980s are told repeatedly that things have improved, in that few people are hungry. Thus older people in Granada contrasted the old days with modern plenty: in the past, especially the years before 1956, shortage of food is central to the stories: 'Heaven was a pinch of sugar, a scrap of meat, an egg' (Slater, 1990: 162). A man in his 50s recalled stealing a loaf: 'I still feel bad about it, but I was so hungry' (p. 163). Another man said:

> Today my nephew asks my mother for a snack of bread and jam, and she wants to know what kind of jam he wants: peach, grape, orange? But in that time when Leopoldo went about Granada begging, what child dared dream of jam? What an idea! Why, there was no bread!

> (p. 164)

FOOD AS A SYMBOL

When I was a PhD student in Edinburgh a friend, Charles Jones, now a professor in Canada, mentioned one day that he missed his mother's cooking, especially her liver and bacon. My family too had had liver and bacon as a regular winter dish, so I offered to cook the dish for him. I casseroled the liver and bacon as it was prepared in my family and served it to Charles. He cleared his plate and said: 'That was delicious but it lacks the Oedipal flavour.'

Years later, I learned that his mother did not casserole her liver and bacon, but grilled them, so my attempt was hopelessly 'wrong'. Even if it had been 'right', however, it would have lacked that Oedipal flavour – food from our families, our childhood, our homeland, our first foreign holiday, is irrevocably fixed for us as special. Our beliefs about food are usually unexamined and buried deep within ourselves. If you are a British or American reader there is one simple test of this – imagine you are walking down a street of a Belgian town looking for somewhere to eat. Can you go into a restaurant which displays a horse's head outside it?

The importance of such feelings cannot be underestimated. Take these examples. First here is Elizabeth David on holiday with a French family near Caen in Normandy in the 1930s.

> The only vivid memory I have of the food in this peaceful and pretty house with its old-fashioned kitchen garden is of tasting mussels for the first time. They were served in a thick creamy

sauce which no doubt had cider or white wine in its composition
. . . To this day a dish of mussels is one of the first things I ask
for upon landing in Northern France, and the last thing I eat
before crossing the channel to return to England, for . . .
although since that first time I have eaten mussels served in
dozens of different ways . . . they never seem to have quite the
cachet, the particular savour, of those mussels of Normandy.

(1964: 30)

Now here is Claudia Roden, an Egyptian Jew:

I was a schoolgirl in Paris then. Every Sunday I was invited together
with my brother and a cousin to eat *ful medames* with some relatives.
This meal became a ritual. Considered in Egypt to be a poor man's
dish, in Paris the little brown beans became invested with all the
glories and warmth of Cairo, our home town, and the embodi-
ment of all that for which we were homesick.

(1970: 11)

For Elizabeth David, then, Normandy is evoked by mussels, and for
Claudia Roden, Cairo by *ful medames*, a little brown bean. For a
Finn, it would be *lakka* (cloudberries) or *puolukka* (cranberries) or
mustikka (bilberries) or reindeer meat.

Food carries the history of the country or region, whether its
modern inhabitants realise it or not. Take Spain:

One wonders what in fact the people of the Iberian Peninsular
originally ate – for olives and garlic were brought by the
Romans; and saffron, black pepper, nutmeg, lemons, cane
sugar, rice and bitter oranges came with the Arab conquerors;
the sweet orange was introduced through Portugal from China;
while the taste for *garbanzos* (chick peas) came with Cartha-
ginians. And it was not until the discovery of America that
Spain, and through her, Europe, first enjoyed potato, tomato,
pimento and chocolate.

(Gili, 1963: 10–11)

Similarly, David points out that the food in the Alsace region of
France is recognisably affected by its history:

The cookery here is very interesting, with a variety of traditional
dishes remarkable even for a French province. This is partly
due, no doubt, to the tenacity with which the people clung to
their old customs during the years of German domination,

partly also because of the influence of an old-established Jewish colony whose traditional dishes . . . have become part of Alsatian cookery.

(David, 1964: 40)

Food also carried its symbolic messages out from Europe with colonial invaders in the past, and with tourists today. A story from West Africa illustrates the colonial point. A Nigerian higher degree student in Cardiff was a lecturer in a teacher training college at home. He had been to a conference for lecturers in teacher training from all the West African countries, including those which had been colonised by France. The meeting took place in a former French colony and at lunchtime the organiser announced that as a great treat the main dish was roast horse. All the delegates from former French colonies beamed and headed for the dining hall, while all those from the ex-British colonies felt repulsed and went out to look for something they could eat. As my student commented, this was purely a legacy of colonialism. None of the people present came from cultures which, before European conquest, had any tradition about horses: the labelling of the horse as 'food' or 'not food' was an inheritance of their former colonial rulers.

Today tourists carry food symbolism with them across Europe, so that hotels in Cyprus offer a breakfast buffet of cheese and ham for the Scandinavians, Germans and Dutch, Spanish resorts serve tea with cow's milk in it for British people; and British hotels offer 'hash browns' at breakfast for the Americans.

FOOD AND TIME

Food and mealtimes are an important part of the daily, weekly, monthly, seasonal and annual cycle, and foods are used to mark special occasions – both regular feasts (such as Christmas or the end of Ramadan) and life-cycle events such as births, marriages and deaths. As Mary Douglas puts it:

Between breakfast and the last nightcap, the food of the day comes in an ordered pattern. Between Monday and Sunday, the food of the week is patterned again. Then there is the sequence of holidays and fast days through the year, to say nothing of life cycles of feasts, birthdays and weddings.

(Douglas, 1975: 251)

Imagine a day in Madrid:

> Breakfast is often no more than a token breaking of the fast, and
> consists of coffee, or thick chocolate, which is: 'the favourite
> drink of the church and allowable even on fast days', into which
> bread, fresh or fried, may be dipped. Lunch is eaten between
> one and four o'clock (in Madrid it is particularly late), allowing
> time for a *siesta* afterwards, a necessity where the midday sun is
> not conducive to work. It consists of a soup, or hors-d'oeuvre, a
> vegetable (which is always served separately before the meat or
> fish course), pasta or rice dish followed by fish or meat, which
> may be accompanied by potatoes. then comes a sweet, and fruit.
> If cheese is offered, it is most likely to be one made from goat's
> milk, or an excellent one called *manchego*, from La Mancha,
> which is a ewe's milk cheese. Wine is drunk at all meals; even the
> children drink it diluted. Between four and nine, or nine-thirty,
> when the evening meal is eaten, there is no official break,
> though tea (at about 6 p.m.) for children usually consists of a
> slice of bread and a bar of chocolate. The Spaniard, who
> finished work at about 7 p.m., can return slowly home, by way of
> aperitifs and talk with his friends, to the evening meal which in
> form resembles lunch.
>
> (Gili, 1963: 9–10)

The food of a northern country also marks out the day. Consider
Crewe's (1980: 181) summary of a day's food in the Netherlands.

> The Dutch maintain that they eat only one meal a day. Break-
> fast, of course, does not count and will consist only of cheese,
> ham, salami, eggs, possibly a steak, rolls and jam, chocolate
> vermicelli and other such fripperies. You can have a full lunch,
> but many restaurants serve what is called *koffietafel* (coffee table)
> with nothing more than soup, a few prawns, meat croquettes, a
> bit of cold ham, beef, chicken or pork, a pâté, some pumper-
> nickel and a little currant bread rounded off with some cheese
> and fruit . . . The real meal of the day is dinner, which they eat
> early compared with other European nations. (Well, they are
> hungry, poor things, with only little snacks all day.)

Crewe is obviously teasing the Dutch here, but the rhythm of the
day is still clear.

The week may be marked by different foods on different days, so
the food item and day are inextricably linked. When Elizabeth David

was living, in the 1930s, with a French family in Paris, Catholics were still required to avoid meat on Fridays, so Friday meant fish. Not even well-cooked fish but: 'the boiled salt cod which was the regular Friday lunch. Grey, slimy, in great hideous flakes, it lay plonked on the plate' (David, 1964: 28). Presumably, the awfulness of this was part of the religious penance. In Finland, Tuesday was pea soup day: that is, the soup of the day in a Finnish restaurant was always *herne keitto* on Tuesdays. In Britain 'Sunday lunch' is a shorthand for describing a particular meal, of roast meat, roast and boiled potatoes, a green vegetable and a second vegetable of another colour, all smothered in gravy (see Murcott, 1982).

Seasons will have their own foods, which mark out the rhythm of the year. For over a thousand years this was because foods were seasonal: some things grew in the summer, some in the autumn, some in winter. Harvest time, lambing, the start of the hen's laying season, the arrival of the first new fruit of summer and so on were the determinants of diet. Fish could only be caught when the sea was calm enough to sail out of the harbour, or when they swam up the local river. Today in much of Europe traditional methods of preserving food (salting it, smoking it and pickling it) have been supplemented or supplanted by tinning, freezing, freeze-drying and irradiating. Then there are imports of out-of-season foods from other regions of the world and a new style of agri-business which ensures supplies of many foods (such as eggs) throughout the year. However, there are still many countries and regions in which seasons are marked by particular foods or dishes, especially for those who live in the countryside and actually grow the food. Take the Tuscan household studied by Calabresi (1987: 122–123):

> In October Adorno and Maria go about their farm in shirtsleeves, picking the last fruit from the trees . . . The warmth of the season increases the pleasure of bringing in the fruit . . . Pears, apples, figs, late peaches and the grapes are warm to the touch on vines and branches; dessert is festooned about the farm.
>
> Fruit, in all its forms, is the luxury of the farm . . . Adorno and Maria eat fruit sparingly, to make it last as long as possible, yet many meals at the end of the winter are finished without it. Few apples remain after March and there is a gap until the May strawberries and the apricots and cherries of June . . .

In Mallorca, ordinary people go out in autumn to gather fungi in the woods, and to search for the edible snails. In the early autumn

Finnish markets are colourful with the piles of red, yellow and purple berries. In Belgium late spring is the time for a stew of baby eels and sorrel; in Finland the summer means crayfish are in season, in the early summer the shad swims up the Loire so local people can eat it grilled with sorrel sauce, and in October there are new walnuts in Greece to cook hare in walnut sauce. In Germany:

> The asparagus season from May to June is treated very seriously
> . . . Many restaurants make a great production of it and whole
> families embark on special excursions to such places to sample
> the new crop.
>
> (Crewe, 1980: 100)

In the highlands of Sardinia, shearing means a feast, for men from several families combine to deal with each man's flock in turn, and are given a big supper afterwards.

> In 1982 at one shearing in Ollolai there were over one hundred
> guests. All were fed roast lamb, boiled mutton, blood pudding,
> ravioli, bread, cheese, olives and copious amounts of wine.
>
> (Berger, 1986: 374)

Festivals will have their own food patterns, too: 'Special foods, such as "wedding cakes" or "roast turkey and cranberry sauce" have special easily recognised associations with particular occasions' (Leach, 1976: 60). In Britain, Christmas means turkey, Brussels sprouts, Christmas pudding and mince pies, but elsewhere in Europe, the Christians celebrate the same festival with very different foods. In many countries, the centre-piece of the dinner is fish. In Norway the traditional Christmas Eve dish was *Whelks tersk*, a whole young cod boiled and served with hollandaise sauce; in Poland the meal was *barszcz*, a soup with boletus mushrooms and beetroot, followed by a whole carp; this carp dish could also be found in parts of Germany:

> Simmered in a beer-flavoured stock and served with a sauce
> including cake crumbs, spices, almonds and dried fruits. The
> fish is not descaled before cooking and it is customary for each
> diner to save a few scales from the carp as a good luck charm for
> the coming year. In Austria the Christmas Eve carp is sliced,
> dipped in egg and breadcrumbs, fried and served with potato
> salad and lemon.
>
> (Crewe, 1980: 93)

The other German Christmas dish was goose 'served with red cabbage and potato dumplings. The stuffing usually contains apples and onions and possibly raisins and nuts' (Crewe, 1980: 98).

In Greece Christmas means *Kourabiedes*, a type of shortbread in the shape of a diamond or a crescent with a clove stuck in it to remind the eater of the spices brought by the Three Kings to the manger. In Germany and Austria the equivalent is *Lebkuchen*, spiced honey cakes, sometimes gilded, and often in ornate shapes. In Denmark both New Year's Eve and Twelfth Night have a special cake. New Year's Eve means 'destiny cake' with three charms hidden in it: a ring, a thimble and a coin. (The three finders will fall in love, not marry and become rich.) Then there is the traditional cake for Twelfth Night (6 January in the Catholic and Protestant churches). A feast of a traditional kind would start with onion soup, then crescent-shaped sausage rolls, vol-au-vents with mushrooms and liver pâté, biscuits with a caraway-seed flavoured smoked curd cheese, and the *Hellig Tre Konger Kage*. This cake has one whole almond in it, and whoever gets that nut is the 'king' for the meal.

There are festivals in the Greek Orthodox calendar unfamiliar to Roman Catholics and Protestants, and these can call for special foods. In Asi Gonia St Basil's day (1 January) is the occasion for *Koliva* (boiled wheatgerm, sweets, sugar, cinnamon and perfume) which is offered to the souls of the dead, or *vassilopitta* (St Basil's pies) (Machin, 1983). On Donoussa (Connell, 1980: 59)

> On the Feast of the Elevation of the Cross (September 14th) the ancient cross of Stavros church on Donoussa was brought outside on a bed of basil to be revered by the congregation. After the service, all the loaves which had been baked and brought in by villagers to be blessed were taken outside, cut into hunks and served with wine and sweetmeats.

The Islamic people living in Europe keep a different religious calendar, with a month (*ramadan*) in which everyone able-bodied should fast from dawn to dusk. Once darkness falls a feast can be eaten, but the devout will not eat, or drink, or even swallow their own saliva for the 10, 12 or even 16 hours of daylight. Europe's Jews will be keeping their religious calendar with their foods alongside those of other faiths.

Life-cycle events such as baptisms, weddings and funerals also imply food of particular kinds. It is only a 'proper' funeral, or wedding or christening if the 'right' foods are served. In a society like Britain, where different social classes have different diets and prefer different food and drink, this shows up in meals served to celebrate weddings. The example which follows shows the 'messages' carried by menus and illustrates how things we take for granted are actually worth studying in some detail.

THE WEDDING MEAL

This section summarises an analysis (Delamont, 1983) of the advice given to brides and their mothers about appropriate food for weddings by the mass media, wedding etiquette books and commercial caterers. The studies of actual weddings (Leonard, 1980; Charsley, 1991) show that different social classes choose to follow different types of advice, which are contrasted in this analysis.

According to the magazines and books, there are two choices of cook: the bride's mother, or a paid outsider, the caterer. There are three possible locations: the bride's family home (house or garden), a public hall, or a commercial club, hotel or restaurant. A paid, non-family, caterer may provide the meal in any of these three types of location: the bride's mother cannot cook in the commercial setting. Figure 2.1 shows the possible cook/setting combinations. All the magazines and advice manuals assume the wedding is for meat-eating people who are not Jewish, Muslim,

Location
Private

Bride's mother	Caterer
Bride's home	Bride's home

Motive

Food provision
for
love   Money

Bride's mother	Caterer
Hired hall	Hotel/restaurant

Public

Figure 2.1 Location and motive

Hindu or Buddhist; there is nothing in the magazines for the family whose daughter is marrying someone of another cuisine.

The decisions about who provides the food, and where it is served, affect the menu, the number of guests and the cost, and are affected by them. The mass media 'experts' are divided about whether or not it is a 'good thing' for the bride's mother to do the cooking. The data we have suggest that the option in the bottom right of Figure 2.1, a public reception where food is provided for money, is the most popular. However, the women's magazines regularly propose menus which the bride's mother can cook herself, which can be contrasted with the commercial menus offered by hotels and caterers. The comparison shows that two very different messages about women's roles are being carried by the meals.

All suggested menus for wedding lunches to be provided by the bride's mother traced are similar. Table 2.1 shows the basic structure of the lunch menus suggested by a variety of magazines and cookery books, from the 1915 edition of Mrs Beeton up to 1980s magazines. While Mrs Beeton's menus are more lavish, the basic structure of the wedding lunch has remained remarkably stable for a century. There may be a soup/fruit juice/melon course before the fish, and the number and variety of vegetables vary, but the basic menu is clearly:

1 Salmon/lobster	4 Wedding cake
2 Poultry	5 Cake and champagne
3 Light pudding (fresh fruit, aerated dish)	6 Coffee and/or tea

All are cold meals, and a luxury food – salmon or lobster – features in many of them. The magazines and cookery books share a common idea of an 'ideal' wedding lunch.

However, this was not what the real couples getting married in Swansea in the late 1960s or in Glasgow in the early 1980s (Charsley, 1991) actually had in their hotels, or other commercial establishments. Leonard (1980: 182) gives a typical menu as follows:

1 Sherry	4 Pears and ice cream
2 Soup	5 Coffee
3 Roast turkey with bacon rolls, roast and mashed potatoes, peas, bread sauce	6 Sherry and wedding cake

Table 2.1 Magazine and cookery book suggestions for a wedding lunch

Source	Suggested guest nos	Hot or cold	1st/fish course	2nd/meat course	Pudding
Woman's Journal August 1981	25	C	Salmon	Chicken	Fruit flan
Wedding Day Summer 1981	8	C	Salmon	Chicken	Trifle, meringues
Woman & Home June 1981	30	C	Salmon	Chicken	Gateaux, fruit salad
Living April 1972	40	C	Smoked salmon	Chicken	Gateaux
Women's Realm May 1980	50	C	Melon	Pork, chicken	Savarin, meringues
Good Housekeeping Cookery Book	–	C	Salmon	Chicken	Gateaux
	–	C	melon	mixed cold meat	lemon soufflé
	–	H	Hot lobster, vol au vents	turkey	lemon chiffon
Woman April 1982	60	C	Smoked salmon	Turkey	Chocolate sponge
Mrs Beeton 1915 edition	?	C	Oyster, sole, turbot, salmon, lobster	Chicken, turkey, lamb, veal, pigeon, beef, foie gras	Fruit creams, meringue, ices

This menu is more like those offered by hotels to enquirers in the 1980s and those in Heaton's (1975) etiquette book, than those in the general magazines and cookery books. Heaton was a hotel manager, and one of his five specimen menus for a reception in a hotel or restaurant is shown in Table 2.2, along with some menus

Table 2.2 Commercial menus

Source	Starter	Main course	Pudding	Coffee?
Heaton 1	Tomato soup	Roast chicken, bread sauce, potatoes, sprouts, carrots	Peach Melba	Yes
Labroke Beef Menu 4 (£7.00)	Melon	Roast beef, sprouts, parsnips, roast potatoes	Profiteroles	Yes
Chicken Menu 9 (£6.00)	Soup	Chicken supreme, peas, carrots, potatoes	Sherry trifle	Yes
Turkey Menu 12 (£6.50)	Tomato soup	Roast turkey, sprouts, carrots, roast potatoes	Gateau	Yes

from Ladbroke's Hotels with 1981 prices. Table 2.2 shows that menus like those served to Leonard's and Charsley's sample are typical of 'catered' public receptions. They are also proper, cooked dinners (assuming there is gravy) as analysed by Murcott (1982). They could not be provided by the bride's mother (unless she missed the ceremony) because they are served hot and demand constant and last minute attention. The proper dinner is what the bride's mother would/should/does provide on other 'special' occasions – e.g. Christmas – but cannot on the wedding day. So she either provides a different kind of special meal in the home *or* her cooking is delegated to a professional who provides a proper dinner away from the bride's home.

There are two different kinds of wedding lunch which can be represented as in Table 2.3. This gives us two different ideal types, one where strange food served in familiar surroundings marks the 'special' occasion, the other where a 'strange' location is familiarised by the 'proper' food, albeit a celebratory kind of proper food. If we repeat Figure 2.1 with the food types added, we get Figure 2.2.

Table 2.3 Two ideal types of wedding lunch

Location	Cook	Temperature	Posture	Meal type
Home	Bride's mother	Cold	Stand	Unusual food
Hotel	Caterer	Hot	Sit	'Proper dinner'

Location
Private

Bride's mother
Bride's home
Cold buffet

Caterer's
Bride's home
?

Motive

Food provision
for love

A   B
C   D

Money

Bride's mother
Hired hall
Cold buffet

Public

Caterer
Hotel, etc.
'Proper dinner'

Figure 2.2 Location, motive and food types

Leonard (1980: 2) comments:

> If white weddings are alive and well in the second half of the twentieth century, it is not because they are outdated charades, but rather because they make important statements about, among other things, the nature of marriages and family relations.

The two types of reception – in terms of location and food – have to be seen in this way. What is being transmitted is a statement about proper food and the proper role of women. At the wedding reception the bride's family are both despatching the bride into a new family unit and demonstrating what kind of people they are. Receptions show the groom, his kin and the guests what lifestyle the bride has and therefore what she should be entitled to in future. That far the two kinds of reception are similar. Both cost money, and show that the bride's father can afford to provide a good meal. But the bride is about to become responsible for feeding the groom so it is also important to show what kind of food her upbringing has led her to treat as proper. The two kinds of reception symbolise this transfer – from a girl who is cooked for, to a woman who does the cooking – in different ways.

The hotel-based 'proper' dinner conveys two clear messages. First the bride's family know what a proper meal looks like, therefore the bride does, and therefore she can and will provide proper dinners for her new husband (Murcott, 1982, 1983). The second 'message' is that – because this meal is in a public place outside the home – the bride is no longer entitled to have meals cooked for her by her mother in her natal home. The phase of 'keeping close and spoiling' so well described by Leonard (1980) is over, and this is captured by the last financial indulgence which is not accompanied by domestic labour from the parents.

Leonard's sample saw a commercial reception as necessary for a proper wedding. Registry weddings did not have a hotel reception, and meals cooked by 'mum' were second best. Magazines which advocate a stylish home reception challenge hotel domination by offering a different message. The bride's mother is *Superwoman*, a cool, calm, collected hostess with organising ability and technological resources (such as freezer, mixer and microwave) (cf. Murcott, 1983). She saves money for her husband by catering herself, and displays that she is a better cook than the professionals. This reception shows the world (and the groom) that the bride has been raised by, and hence will be, the perfect hostess, the highly organised wife. Only a family in good housing will contemplate a reception from home *from choice* so the financial standing of the bride's father is displayed by the setting of the reception, against which the home-produced food is a kind of 'symbolic' economy, negated by the expensive food items in it. To summarise: the message system of the two kinds of wedding reception is that 'traditional working class' and 'middle-class superwoman' have produced two rather different kinds of bride. (See Delamont, 1983, for further details of this analysis.)

Similar analyses can be done of appropriate food for funerals, for christenings, for wedding anniversary parties and so on. The lifecycle occasion is only properly marked if the correct food is served.

FOOD AND RELIGION

Food is also inextricably linked to religious beliefs, practices and identities. Muslims and Jews should avoid pork, Catholics were asked to avoid meat on Fridays and in Lent until the Second Vatican Council in the early 1960s, the Greek Orthodox family Easter is celebrated by a lamb and so on. Chapter 8 is all about religion, but here it is important to stress that a person's most cherished beliefs and sense of identity may be embodied in *not* eating certain foods, or by eating them on specific occasions, or by serving them on particular days.

The next theme in this chapter is that of drinks and drinking. Here all the symbolic, religious and other features of food apply again.

DRINKS AND DRINKING

Alongside food, drink is also symbolic. Anthropologists have paid relatively little attention to drink, as Douglas (1987) pointed out. There were all sorts of findings about drink buried in their publications, but it did not feature as interesting in its own right, the way burial rites or betrothal ceremonies did.

Here three themes will be briefly mentioned: drinks as national or regional symbols, drinks as 'markers' of social relations and drinks as 'markers' of gender roles. Drinks are just as symbolic of different nations or cultures as food is. Two examples of this will suffice: 'Most Finns, in public, seem to drink buttermilk with meals, and quantities of weakish coffee at other times' (Crewe, 1980: 191). Buttermilk is very much a drink of Germany and Scandinavia: not of the south. In contrast men in Greece also drink quantities of coffee but it is anything but weak: Greek coffee is very strong and very thick, served in tiny cups with a glass of water. Greeks do not drink buttermilk.

Just as older people can remember when food was short, and when rye bread was the only food, so too there are memories of drinks that today are commonplace being luxuries. In the Swiss village studied by Netting (1981: 37): 'Adults remember when coffee was only for Sundays or feast days, and the elderly recall a time when coffee was a special treat reserved for Christmas Eve'. What a person chooses to drink is as much a part of their national and cultural identity, the seasons, the life cycle and religion as what they eat. The paper by Thornton (1987) on *schnapps* and *sekt* in an Austrian village is a good example of unpicking the symbolism of drink within one community. In the farming area in the Austrian countryside there were few 'rules' and little significance attached to non-alcoholic drinks. Fruit juices were given to children and drunk by adults mixed with mineral water, as are carbonated commercial drinks. Water, either from the tap or bottled, was rarely drunk except for health reasons. Lots of coffee was drunk throughout the day, with tea as an occasional substitute. All these drinks were *not* symbolically loaded. The symbolically important drinks were of two kinds, both alcoholic: *schnapps* and *sekt* headed the two categories. *Schnapps* (which comes in many colours and flavours) is a brandy-like drink: that is a fortified 'wine'. It can be bought in shops but many people made their own which was considered better. *Schnapps* is drunk in informal gatherings of intimates or with *new* friends to signify the growing intimacy. *Sekt*, which is a fizzy wine, is bought from shops, and is drunk on formal and traditional occasions, such as birthdays and anniversaries, town or village holidays, or national holidays especially New Year's Eve and Shrove Tuesday (*Fasching*). Austria has many big dances held in public halls, and these would be *sekt* affairs too. Thus, for the Austrians Thornton studied, the pouring of a glass of *schnapps* or *sekt* marked two quite distinct types of social event.

In many societies the divisions between men and women are marked by what it is acceptable for them to drink. In traditional British and Irish culture respectable women did not go into pubs or bars at all, and even when this has vanished, many drinks are clearly labelled as 'masculine' or 'feminine'. At the time of writing a beer commercial in Britain includes a man asking for a 'snowball' and the faces of watching men reveal this is *not* a drink for a 'real' man. The hero then adds that he wants a beer for himself, and his male audience are able to relax. In Britain, drinks with names like 'snowball' are clearly marked as 'female'.

In some cultures neither sex is supposed to drink alcohol (all Muslims should be teetotal, as traditionally were Methodists and the stricter Scottish non-conformist sects). In others men drink alcohol and women do not, or rather respectable women do not. Gurr (1987: 233):

In Maigret's Paris men drink and women don't. Both the two women who drink too much do not report a murder. And of the three men who are abnormal because they do *not* drink, two are murderers.

Simenon started the Maigret books in 1930, and they describe a Paris of the 1930s. (The time does not change, so that the 1940s, 1950s and 1960s never happened.) Gurr uses the 102 stories to construct a world structured by drinks. Drinks mark class and national identities, but also gender. Noticeably, Gurr comments, Madame Maigret never drinks alcohol in the stories, only coffee and a verbena *tisane.* Cowan (1991) maps the respectable drinks among the Greeks in Sohos. Women drink coffee very sweet (*ghliko*), men's coffee is served less sweet. Women drink their wine *imighliko* (sweet and mild) while men prefer the *brusko* (harsh and manly). Men drink ouzo (with olives), while women drink *yinekio* (syrupy mint and fruit flavoured brandies). Similarly in the Breton community studied by Maryon McDonald (1989), men drink rough red wine while women drink coffee, or tea if they are aping Parisian manners, for tea is higher status than coffee among these rural Bretons.

The final theme in this chapter is food preparation as *work.* Laments for the loss of traditional foods ignore the back-breaking labour involved in making them, which usually fell on women.

FOOD PREPARATION AS WORK

Many writers bemoan the loss of traditional national and regional food. However it is important to recognise that many traditional dishes involved much labour and many hours. In the highlands of Corsica bread was made from chestnut flour, involving the collection of nuts, shelling and boiling them, grinding the nuts to flour, then making dough and then baking bread. In the Sardinian village studied by Berger (1986: 364)

> Many women still participate in multi-household work groups preparing *pane caresau.* The work is not as laborious or time consuming as in the past, since the dough is mixed and prepared in a commercial bakery. But it still involves 6–8 women working an entire day, dawn to dusk, to produce enough bread to supply a single household for 1–2 months. Labour is exchanged on a reciprocal basis.

It is no surprise that women now choose commercially baked wheat bread when they can afford it and get hold of it. Connell (1980) contains many accounts of the hard work involved in food production by traditional methods on Amorgos. In the French Basque community of Sainte-Engrâce, the women regarded the pig-killing season as 'the bad month' (Ott, 1981: 36) because of the mess, the smells and the 'numerous unpleasant tasks' they had to do. Men killed the pigs, but women had to clean the intestines, cook the meat, make pâté, black puddings, terrine, *confit de porc*, spiced sausages; and cure the bacon and ham with salt and red pepper. These tasks took a woman and a relative (such as a sister-in-law) three days, and were essential but distasteful. Ott found that if she helped women with this task they felt able to talk to her about intimate matters, because it was such awful work she had demonstrated her commitment to them by participating in it. No outsider would be surprised if a woman wanted to buy her ham in a shop after seeing domestic pig killing and food preparation.

The burden on women is not the only reason for the 'loss' of traditional foods, of course. Traditional foods may vanish because they are associated with poverty, or because women are no longer willing to spend time on them, or both. In the Breton village studied by McDonald (1989) wholemeal bread was not available because it reminded the villagers of the peasant food of the past. When she wanted it, McDonald had to drive to a town where it was sold to the middle classes.

CONCLUSIONS

Throughout this chapter the symbolic importance of food and drink has been stressed. Once that is understood, the passions aroused by policies made in Brussels become clear. If the British are attached to sausages that are 50 per cent bread, then directives about changing their content are an attack not only on the sausage, but on our taken-for-granted understanding of the world.

SUGGESTED READING/ACTIVITY

Read Jane Grigson's (1983) *European Cookery* and look at the pictures. Compare the chapters on Greece and Scandinavia, focusing on the fats used, the seasonings, the vegetables and fruits. Cook a dish from a cuisine strange to you, or a whole meal from an unfamiliar country.

Chapter 3

The vines that trail
Farming and fishing in western Europe

> The fruits that dangle and the vines that trail . . .
>> (Flecker, 1947: 18)

INTRODUCTION

The Common Agricultural Policy (CAP) and the Common Fisheries Policy (CFP) are central to the EEC and thus to all of western Europe. There are useful books about their origins and development (e.g. Clout, 1984; Hill, 1984; and Wise, 1984) and they are not discussed in detail here. Like the book as a whole this chapter is focused at the micro-level: it is about the life of a fisherman putting out from a harbour in Brittany, a shepherd moving sheep up and down the mountains of rural Greece and a farmer growing potatoes in Ayrshire or grapes in Portugal or olives in Spain.

There are three main sections, moving from the most dangerous occupation (fishing), through pastoralism (herding animals) to farming. The type of fisherman, animal herder or farmer who has been studied by anthropologists has largely been the small-scale worker. Research on farmers, for example, has been concentrated on 'peasant' farmers – people producing mixed crops mainly to feed themselves. There is less observational material on those involved in agri-businesses (but see Newby, 1977) than on peasants such as Eloi and Eulalia, the Portuguese couple studied by Jenkins (1979). The word 'peasant' is itself very problematic, and has been defined and redefined by scholars for fifty years. Here it is used to mean any family whose farming is predominantly to feed themselves, rather than to sell. In the 1990s 'peasants' in Europe are increasingly elderly, partially dependent on pensions or benefits, and may be the last of their kind. However, scholars have predicted the end of the 'peasant' for years (e.g. Franklin, 1969; Mendras, 1970; Bailey, 1971b) and it is equally possible that urban unemployment may send people back to a rural existence where at least they eat. 'Peasant' has negative connotations in English, implying stupidity, backwardness and ignorance. It is *not* used in that sense here, merely as a shorthand for a subsistence family-based farming.

Before the detailed material on fishing, herding and farming, the basic issue of regional inequalities needs to be sketched. Clout (1984) emphasises how variably settled Europe is, in that some countries and regions (e.g. Belgium and the Paris basin) are settled densely while other areas are sparsely populated (e.g. western Ireland, the Mani peninsula of Greece). Hill's (1984) companion volume is an excellent account of regional inequalities. Hamburg, the richest area in the EEC, has inhabitants who are on average five times better off than an average inhabitant of Calabria in southern Italy and twelve times better off than the poorest Portuguese.

CAP AND CFP

> Disputes over who should fish what and where seem to stir national emotions far more than dour problems associated with, for example, the production of cars or steel, despite the greater economic importance of the latter.
>
> (Wise, 1984: 1)

> In the early days of the Community the CAP was perceived as a move towards the integration of its member states; it was the first major common policy. There is no doubt that in the past decade it has become a force for disintegration.
>
> (Hill, 1984: 157)

When the CAP began, the hunger of the war years was a vivid memory for the Belgian, Dutch, German, French and Italian delegates who agreed to it. Also, the majority of farmers of those countries – that is the majority of those who had votes – were peasant farmers, not owners of large, agri-business farms. It was a policy designed to prevent anyone starving, and to help the producer with a few cows and a couple of pigs on an unmechanised small family farm.

Hill (1984: 20) points out that when the CAP began, in 1958, over 15 million people (over 20 per cent of the working population) were dependent on farming for their income. The original six countries (Italy, Germany, The Netherlands, Belgium, Luxembourg and France) had very different agricultural policies, and a great many types of soil, climate and crops were involved. The CAP had the aims of increasing productivity and modernising farming, getting farmers a decent living, stabilising food markets, assuring supplies of food, and getting the food to consumers at reasonable prices. The idea was to allow food and drink to move freely between countries, and to equalise prices for agricultural products. Over the ten years from 1958 progress was made towards these goals.

The famous problem associated with the CAP, other than its costs, is surpluses. Originally the idea was to smooth out seasonal fluctuations in food prices and stop anyone starving because a food had run out – so the EEC buy up food when there is a glut and store it, to stop prices dropping, and then release the food when it is scarcer to stop prices rocketing up. When the CAP began, Hill (1984: 35) points out, all the six countries had to import food, and they all hoped that the CAP would make the community self-sufficient. It was *so* successful that soon the surpluses built up too much. This was partly because everyone began having smaller families so the population of the EEC did not grow. By the late 1960s political pressures were building up to change the system, and the accession of Denmark, Ireland and Great Britain meant that the CAP faced new strains, followed by even more difficulties when Greece, Spain and Portugal were added. Hill is convinced that the CAP is distorting the EEC by using too great a proportion of its budget, and that the 'dumping' of surpluses disturbs the world food market. Hill (1984: 117) concludes:

> The failure of the CAP is comprehensive. It has totally failed to improve the relative position of the agricultural population even on average. Within this it has benefited the rich farmers and regions, rather than the poor, largely at the expense of the consumers, the poorer bearing the major burden because they are both more numerous and spend a higher proportion of their income on food.

This chapter is about the poor farmers who have not benefited from the CAP, rather than the rich ones who have.

The Common Fisheries Policy has been politically important in the development of the EEC. Norway, for example, voted not to join in the 1970s because of the CFP. Wise (1984: 1) points out:

The image of brave, individualistic fishermen hunting for food in an often hostile environment seems to attract more sympathy than those conjured up by the mass-production of metal or motor-vehicles.

Wise (1984: Chapter 2) contains a useful discussion of the fishing industries in all the western European countries, with maps of fishing grounds and explanations of where fish of different types are caught. The section on The Netherlands (pp. 37–38) is useful background reading to the paper by van Ginkel (1991). As with agriculture, countries are concerned about the availability of fish as food and about the jobs in the fishing industry. However, unlike farming, fish are a 'natural' resource and can be exhausted by over-fishing. So fishing policy is concerned with balancing fish stocks and national interests. The CFP was re-negotiated in the 1970s and a new CFP was agreed in 1983.

The CFP is difficult to understand because a lot of different issues are involved. The ideas behind it are to regulate which fishing grounds are open to the boats of which nations, to conserve fish stocks, to prevent fish prices dropping too low and cheap imports getting into the EEC so fishermen's incomes stay at reasonable levels. At the same time the market for fish may change as people choose to eat it or not, which is related to price, religion, and to taste and fashion. Wise (1984: 212) says that as fish prices rose in the EEC during the 1970s, consumption dropped. The central tension in the EEC fishing disputes is whether all the territorial waters of all the member states are open to all the ships of all the other member nations, or not. It is also very hard to 'police' fishing – especially when catches can be landed at dozens of different ports. In the 1982/83 agreement member nations had fishing territories and quotas for different types of fish – so, for example, Belgium was entitled to take 28,900 tonnes of cod equivalent of the seven major species and Denmark 344,000 (Wise, 1984: 238).

Both Hill and Wise published their analyses a decade ago, and they pre-date the accession of Greece, Spain and Portugal, as well as the reunification of Germany. Both books need to be revised and republished in the light of changes since the enlargement.

FISHING AND FISHING COMMUNITIES

The anthropological literature on fishing and fishing communities is not large. There is Tunstall's (1972) study of trawlermen operating out of Hull. Portugal's fishing communities have been studied by Twig Johnson (1979), Mendonsa (1982), Cole (1991) (and she is unusual in focusing on women, and including a woman skipper in her sample) and Brogger (1990). Salamone (1986) is an ethnography of a Greek island dependent on fishing, van Ginkel (1989, 1991) are studies of oyster and mussel fishermen in The Netherlands, Sanmartin (1982) writes on a Spanish lake fishing community, Pi-Sunyer (1978) on Catalonian fishing, and Jorion (1982) on Houat, a Breton island fishing community.

Salamone's study is useful for highlighting how the annual cycle was measured by the type of fish available:

> Village life passed through five distinct periods of productive activity . . . 1) from March to April was Atlantic mackerel season (*Skoubri*); 2) from the middle of May to the middle of August they fished chub mackerel (*Kolios*); 3) from 15th August to the end of January they fished for a type of anchovy (*Koliaroundia*); 4) during the same period they went out after horse mackerel (*safridia*), sardines (*sardeles*) and anchovies (*hapsia*); 5) from the beginning of August to the end of March it was hornfish (*zarganes*), and sand smelt (*atherinia*); and 6) from September until the end of December they went out for bonito (*palamides*).
>
> (Salamone, 1986: 56)

As boats get larger and safer, fishing communities are less vulnerable to the weather, but fish supplies are often seasonal, and the CFP has imposed periods of non-activity to conserve stocks. So, while other fishing communities would not have the same calendar as Salamone's, all fishing communities do still have a pattern of activities closely related to what can be caught.

Johnson's (1979) fieldwork in a fishing community in the southeast of Portugal (the Algarve) focused on the 116 men who sailed on twenty-seven boats. In Povo da Praia the boats leave between one and five in the morning so that the men are ready to haul in the catch soon after sunrise. It may take as long as two hours or as little as thirty minutes to get to the fishing ground, but as the boats can only get out of the natural harbour at or near low tide, their departure is governed by the tides. Hauling in the nets takes from three to nine hours.

Once the fish are on board the boat, the crew sail to Tavira, the regional capital. On the journey – about forty minutes – the men clean the nets, having removed the fish from them, and have lunch. The fish are sold, the boat takes the nets back to the fishing ground and sets them there, an hour's work. Finally they can go home, after a working day of 7–14 hours. Such traditional fishing is dangerous, dirty, hard work and involves co-operation among groups of men to accomplish.

The tensions between members of the same crew were considerable, and one way to resolve these was the *caldeirada*: a communal meal at the end of the fishing day. A crew gather in a *taberna* or the skipper's house, and share a meal of fish, bread and wine. The profits from the day's fishing are distributed, other crews are 'slagged off' and gossiped about, any complaints about fellow crew members aired in a ritualised way and jokes are told. Cole's (1991) research in Vila Cha – a fishing and farming village north of Oporto – is unusual in that some women there are actually sea-going 'fishermen'. Most European maritime communities have a strict division of labour by sex, in which women stay on land, and men go to sea. Indeed, in many such communities, it is believed to be bad luck for women to go on board fishing boats. However, there are exceptions and Cole reports that 'there are small fisheries in Brittany, Galicia, Sardinia, parts of Ireland, and parts of Sweden where women regularly go fishing with men' (Cole, 1991: 65). Vila Cha women seem to have been more actively involved as sea-going fishermen than in other Portuguese villages:

> they took out fishing liccnccs and wcrc both boat owners and boat skippers; they went greater distances at sea . . . and during the sardine fishing that took place between sunset and sunrise, women stayed out on boats overnight.
>
> (p. 66)

Vila Cha, like other villages on the Atlantic coast of Portugal has a basic division between families who live inland and farm the land (*os lavradores*) and the fishing families who live near the beach (*os pescadores*). In Nazare (Mendonsa, 1982; Brogger, 1990) a tourism and fishing community near Lisbon the farmers are called *pe calcado* (those with shoes) and the fishermen *gente da praia* (people of the beach). In Vila Cha the women from fishing families make a substantial contribution to the family's budget by a back-breaking form of labour, gathering seaweed:

> My first view of the community was on a rainy May morning
> when women were at work on the beach, wading waist-deep in
> the water, collecting seaweed in huge circular hand nets and
> spreading it to dry on the sands.
>
> (Cole, 1991: xv)

Cole argues that women's work was 'indispensable' to the local
fishing economy. Apart from gathering seaweed (which was sold as
fertiliser to *lavradores*), and running the household, they grew the
families' vegetables, did the marketing of the fish, unloaded the
boats, sorted the catch and maintained the nets. This task, before
nylon, was vital and time-consuming. Cotton nets were carried to a
freshwater river, washed clean of salt, carried back to the beach,
spread out to dry, and then re-rolled and delivered back to the
boat. To an outsider the seaweed harvest sounds the hardest work;
the women

> spent long hours on the beach during the summer months.
> They waded in the shallows, often in water up to their necks,
> and harvested the loose seaweed in their hand nets. Or they
> collected the seaweed as it washed onshore with the incoming
> tide. They carried the heavy wet seaweed to the high-water mark
> to be spread on the beach to dry for a few days.
>
> (Cole, 1991: 75)

This is a typical peasant task: exhausting, dirty and smelly.

Fishing by traditional methods was hard work, often at unsocial
hours, for uncertain reward, and could be extremely dangerous.
All the studies of fishing communities recount deaths when men
were lost at sea. Fishing could provide men with immense satisfaction, but it was also desperately demanding. In many fishing
villages, including Cap Lloc in Catalonia and Nazare in Portugal,
dealing with tourists is an easier way to make money (Pi-Sunyer,
1978; Mendonsa, 1982). As demanding as fishing, but without the
same possibilities of going over to tourism, is pastoralism.

PASTORALISM

There are two kinds of animal husbandry of a traditional kind to
be discussed here. (Animal rearing intensively, often indoors as
agri-business, is *not* discussed.) There are places which produce
enough food for the animals to eat close to the village so the

humans can sleep in the same bed all the year round while the animals move around a few pastures within easy reach. Then there are herders who have to engage in transhumance: where the animals have to be moved to summer pastures which are different from winter ones, usually up in mountains that are snow-covered in winter. The humans (either everyone, or merely the able-bodied men) have to go with the animals and camp in huts or tents alongside their flocks. In Mediterranean countries the animals are usually moved because the hot dry summers mean that grazing is found in higher pastures, in Alpine ones the retreat of snow reveals lush grazing, and the lower fields produce hay which keeps the animals going in winter. Friedl's (1974) study of Kippel and Netting's (1981) of Torbel are ethnographies of Swiss Alpine communities where transhumant pastoralism is practised, but crops, notably potatoes, are also grown.

Transhumant peoples are particularly interesting to anthropologists, more so than the stock-rearing villager who lives in his own house all the year round. This section focuses predominantly on the 'heroic' transhumant pastoralists. There are studies of French Basque shepherds (Ott, 1981), of Spanish transhumant cowherds (Freeman, 1979), of Greek mainland shepherds (Campbell, 1964), Cretan shepherds (Herzfeld, 1985), those on Naxos (Stewart, 1991), and Sardinian herdsmen (Berger, 1986; Schweizer, 1988). Rosenberg (1988) is a study of a French Alpine village where cows and sheep are kept, and Rogers (1991) of a sheep-herding village in the Aveyron district of France. The Swiss research is by Friedl (1974) and Netting (1981).

There is less published research on those who move cows around than on shepherds. The hardest lives reported among cow herders are probably those of the Pasiegos (Freeman, 1979) and Vaqueiros (Catedra, 1992) who herd cows in the mountains along the northern coast of Spain. This is the coast of lush meadows, forest, plentiful vegetables, snow-capped mountains, rain, fog and mist. Freeman found the Pasiegos's environment a total contrast to the area of Castile, where she had previously done research (Freeman, 1970).

The Pasiegos, who herd cattle up and down the mountains facing the Atlantic behind Santander, are said by themselves and other Spaniards to be characterised by *recelo*: suspicious reserve. Freeman reports that they felt inferior to and stigmatised by other Spaniards, and marginal to Spanish society. They are one of the *pueblos malditos* or despised peoples along with the Vaqueiros of Asturias, the Margatos of Leon and the gypsies. The Pasiegos inhabit marginal land, suitable only for maize, rye or barley not wheat; raise livestock, and historically used chestnuts as a staple food. (Hence the proverb about the poverty of those who live in the mountains: an estate in the mountains is 'two worms and a chestnut'.) Freeman argues that a transhumant existence (because it involves leaving home where one's reputation is known), trading and commerce, and dealing in animal products (leather and flesh) are all low-status activities in Spain.

The mobility and hardship of a Pasiegos family's life is illustrated by Freeman's case study of Tista Pelayo Maza, his wife and their three children. They moved house twenty times each year between seven 'homes'. Their longest stay is two months in one place, the shortest a week. Families travel light, and only have real furniture in their main home – the *cabana* or *vividora* in the lowest meadow. When Freeman travelled with them, the family took a second set of cutlery for her – normally all five people shared one knife, fork and spoon. In the upper cabins/huts they slept on the hay, and clothing changes were minimised. Children can only reach school when the family is in the lower meadows so they either miss education for much of the year, or live with elderly sedentary relatives in the valley bottom. Unlike the Alpine cowherds (e.g. Friedl, 1974; Netting, 1981; Rosenberg, 1988) abandoning farming and relying on the tourist who wants a skiing holiday in winter or a climbing holiday in summer is not an option in northern Spain.

Shepherds living off herds of sheep (and sometimes goats as well) have been studied more than cow-herding peoples. Berger (1986) is an ethnography of transhumant shepherds in Sardinia, in the highlands known as the Barbagia. 'Normal' transhumant pastoralists spend the winter in the lowlands or valleys and go up to the mountains away from village life in the summer. 'Reverse' transhumant pastoralists 'live' that is, have their home villages – in the mountains and take their animals down to the valleys/lowlands in winter. The shepherds of Ollolai, Berger's village, are of this type. Their home village, where the women, children and elderly people live, is in the mountains, which is too cold for the sheep in winter because there is no shelter and no food. So the men take the flocks down to the lowlands, and live alone alongside their sheep. This is hard work, as sheep have to be milked twice a day, which with a flock of 150–200 ewes is a lot of milking. Then either the milk has to be made into cheese (*fiore sardo*) in the fields or carried to the nearest road to be collected by a lorry. The men are away for eight or nine months of the year, and the only way in which life has got easier in the last twenty years is that trucks are used to transfer them from one pasture to another, rather than being walked along. The village of Ollolai only had enough pasture for a quarter of the sheep owned by the villagers, and then only enough to support them for part of the year. Shearing is a major task: 'shearing is extremely time-consuming and requires much more labour power than the individual shepherds . . . can mobilise within their own families' (Berger, 1986: 372–373).

Ott (1981) reports similar hardships among the French Basque shepherds she studied, in Sainte-Engrâce. Only 376 people now live in Sainte-Engrâce which had a population of over 1,000 in the last century. The men look after 4,000 sheep which are milked for cheese making. The sheep are taken up into the mountains in late May by the able-bodied men, 'who look forward to returning to the mountains and to the exclusively male social world of the herding hut' (1981: 34). The shepherds work in teams, and do not sleep in the mountain huts all the time, but work a duty rota, sharing night duty. As well as guarding the sheep and milking them, the men make mountain cheeses. (During the spring, in the village, men make *etxe-gazna* or house cheeses.) In September the sheep are brought back down from the mountains, for the eight-month winter. In that period the sheep are moved from pasture to pasture up to five times a day. The families also rear pigs and cows. The latter are taken up to the mountains in late June. Apart from animal husbandry the major task is cutting hay (up to three crops each summer) which is back-breaking work for everyone in the community. Among the Sainte-Engrâce shepherds, skill in making mountain cheese is a source of social status: 'Within the neighbourhood or *quartier* the social status of a man depends largely upon the quality of his mountain cheese' (Ott, 1981: 179). Ott gave families Cheddar cheeses as presents, which were discussed avidly and compared with the high-status mountain cheese, the lower-status house cheese and the even lower-status machine-made cheeses, especially cows'-milk ones, available in the town shops.

Ott (1981) provides details of the hardships of the mountain life as did Campbell (1964) in his classic work on the Sarakatsani who move flocks around northern Greece and make feta. Herzfeld's

(1985) Cretan shepherds face equal hardships, though he does not appear to have worked with sheep in the mountains himself. Herding animals is lonely, demands skill and courage, and is physically demanding. Men die in falls trying to rescue animals (see Ott, 1981: 118; Berger, 1986: 385), and vigilance is necessary. Sheep and especially lambs are attacked by animals and get trapped by bad weather or fall into crevices or over cliffs. Ott (1981: 119) reports one man who died 'in the gorge of Ehujarve, when his sheep pressed him to the edge of the precipice as he distributed salt among them'.

In those pastoral cultures where men prove their masculinity not by their cheese but by their skilled animal theft, herding animal involves preventing the sheep from being stolen by other mountain men, proving their masculinity and skill. Herzfeld (1985) and Stewart (1991) are both full of material on how the ability to steal a sheep from the flock of an 'enemy' is the real mark of a man.

Berger's (1986) research shows the Sardinian shepherds' similar attitude to livestock theft. To be *abile* (capable), and to have *balentia* (masculine skill and bravery), is to be a potentially successful thief.

> Young men occasionally undertake small thefts to validate their *balentia*. These are far more than youthful pranks, however, they may help mark the transition from boyhood to manhood, since a boy who has marked himself *abile* is one who can be left alone with the flocks . . . At younger ages boys would sometimes act out these values by stealing cherries or chestnuts.
>
> (Berger, 1986: 227)

Pastoralism is extraordinarily hard work. If the animals have to be fed on hay in the winter, then as well as caring for the animals there is the necessity of getting the hay-making done. If they graze all the year round they have to be moved so they get enough grass. The way of life is only viable as long as enough young fit people will move the animals, and as long as someone will buy the milk, or the meat, or the wool, or the skins or the cheeses. Rosenberg's (1988) village of Abriès had sold all its milk to Nestlés for many years, and its pastoralism was irretrievably destroyed when Nestlé's stopped collecting milk in the region in 1970. Most of the permanent population now live on pensions, and few animals are kept.

Pastoralism has been a way of life for mountain-dwellers in Europe for a thousand years, but it may be doomed. If there is no market for the product, it will only survive if young men want to adhere to the *macho* values of herding, and young women are prepared to keep the home fires burning. Equally threatened by agri-business is peasant farming, the subject of the next section.

FARMING COMMUNITIES

Most of the anthropology of Europe has been focused on people feeding themselves from farming of a subsistence/peasant type. There are few studies of people engaged in agri-business farming (but see Newby, 1977). For every account of someone growing thousands of tons of sugar beet and buying all their own food in a supermarket there are fifty accounts of a peasant household with one cow, three pigs, a few hectares of maize and a vegetable plot.

This section deals with access to land, especially by inheritance, and then focuses on the nature of farmwork, its division of labour, and foreshadows its collapse (which is the main theme of Chapter 5). To understand the everyday lives of people in farming areas, the first important point to grasp is the importance of land, the next the importance of water, and the third the varieties of land. Clearly no-one can grow anything unless they have access to land to plant crops in, but land without water is not useful. In southern Europe rights to water for irrigation may be as important as access to land itself.

'Land' comes in many types, even in one area round one village. Subsistence or peasant farming often depends on having access to several types of land which are used for several different types of crops. In Sicily, for example, a family 'need' some wheat-growing land, an olive grove, some kitchen garden, some grazing land and some space for orange and lemon trees to provide a balanced diet. So, when focusing on studies of farming, types of land for different crops are vital for a family to survive. Davis (1973) conducted a detailed study of land use and farming in a southern Italian town he called Pisticci. The land was used in three distinct ways: the town where houses were built, the land that can be farmed and the wasteland which is useless for farming. Douglass's (1975) study of Basque farming showed a similar division between the homestead, the farm land and pasture land, and the mountain land where bracken and ferns were gathered. In Kippel (Friedl, 1974: 43) there are four types of agricultural land: garden plots (*Garten*), fields planted with potatoes and grain (*Ackerland*), hayfields which can sometimes be grazed after the hay-making (*Wiese*), and land only fit for grazing (*Weide*).

To be a peasant farmer one needs land, of the relevant types, either owned, or rented, or at worst sharecropped. Sharecropping is a system where the sharecropper provides all the labour, and gives the landowner half the crop. This is useful for a landowner who cannot work his or her land, such as elderly widows, but does not lead to investment in the agricultural land. Land ownership can be achieved by purchase, but in most traditional communities land is rarely sold, and the main way to acquire it is through inheritance. The inheritance pattern is one major difference between southern and northern Europe.

The big difference between Pisticci (Davis, 1973) and Echalar and Murelaga (Douglass, 1975), where Pisticci represents southern Europe and Echalar northern Europe, is the way land is passed on from one generation to the next. In southern Italy, Greece and southern Spain it is customary for all the children of a landowner to share the land between them when their parent dies. Land therefore gets split up into tiny portions (although it gets reunited by marriage). In northern Spain, central and northern Italy, Eire, Germany and in Britain, land is *not* divided up in this way. One heir gets the land, the brothers and sisters get other types of property. The fragmentation of land into tiny plots by having multiple heirs has been blamed for the underdevelopment of farming in southern Italy and other parts of southern Europe. Schneider and Schneider (1976: 63) worked in a village in Sicily they called Villamaura. They report how, when a smallholder died, he had five plots of scattered land, to be divided between nine heirs. The land was of three types:

1 an olive grove, 3 kilometres from Villamaura;
2 two plots good enough to grow wheat, each 5 kilometres from Villamaura, but only one on a road;
3 two grazing plots (that is, land fit for animals to forage on) one only 8 kilometres from Villamaura, the other 10 kilometres away, neither on a road and only one on a mule path.

The heirs, as is customary, called in a surveyor to create nine equal shares. He made the tiny olive grove one share, and subdivided the other four plots into eight 'shares'. The nine heirs then drew lots to see which share they would inherit, in public. The heir who drew lot A had to make a cash payment to the other eight heirs because lot A was seen to be more valuable. The eight heirs inherited little bits of wheat land and pasture scattered all over the area. After the lots had been drawn one of the eight accused the heir who had got the olive grove of cheating in collusion with the surveyor. The size of the plots was tiny – one woman owned 231/832 of a plot which was in total *only* 0.05 hectares in size, while a cousin owned the rest.

Similar patterns of fragmentation are found in Greece and Spain. Kenna (pc) had a Greek friend who inherited a fortieth share of an hotel in Kalamata: a more valuable inheritance before the 1986 earthquake in the town than after it! Fraser (1973: 26) interviewed Juan Certes, aged 73, who was a trusted surveyor, called on to divide up inheritances. He describes the skills needed in the hills of Andalusia:

> In this broken and mountainous land you've got to know a lot because its not a matter of dividing the land into so many plots of equal size. It's a question of dividing it into plots of equal production. A plot without water will have to be larger than an irrigated plot or a plot with fruit bearing trees, so that each heir will get the same benefit.

The single-heir system common in northern Spain, and other parts of northern Europe, produces a different pattern. Lison-Tolosana (1976) has described it for Galicia, in the fishing and farming villages, O'Neill (1983) for northern Portugal, and Douglass (1975) explores it in the Basque country. He compared the collapse of farming in one Basque village and its survival in another. Echalar had suffered an exodus of young people, Murelaga had not. Echalar is near the French border and San Sebastian, and had always relied on smuggling for part of its wealth. Murelaga is near Bilbao and Guernica. Echalar has been depopulated and its agriculture has collapsed.

The traditional farming pattern was centred on a homestead – in Basque a *baserria* farmed by a *baserritarra* – which was a large stone building. The ground floor held the livestock and the tools, the first floor was the family's living quarters, and the top storey held the hay loft and stores such as apples. This was an excellent way of using the heat from the animals and the insulating effect of hay to keep the humans warm – but it was smelly and insect-ridden. Each farmstead had three types of land: cereal lands, meadow lands where animals grazed, and mountain lands where ferns were cut for animal bedding and then, when soiled put on the cereal lands for fertiliser.

The domestic group – the *echekoak* – was traditionally a family of three generations. There would be a senior married couple, a junior married couple, and the unmarried children of both. One child in each generation is the heir, the siblings can stay in the *baserria* as long as they are single, but if they marry they must leave and give up all rights to it. The senior couple choose the heir and disinherit their other children – and hand over the farmstead at the heir's marriage.

Because Echalar was near the French border, smuggling was an important source of income. Young men also went to the USA to be shepherds in Nevada and Arizona. In 1966 Douglass found there were twenty-nine men from Echalar working as shepherds in the USA. Young women have, since 1945, also left both the villages, mainly to work in France as hotel maids in tourist areas such as Lourdes. Male and female experiences of migrant labour are very different. Men live and work with other Basque men, or alone, and have no need to learn other languages. Women learn French and Castilian, meet many other people, and no longer want to be an *echekoandria* in Echalar.

Douglass explains the collapse of farming in Echalar, and its survival in Murelaga by contrasting the kinship pattern, the settlement pattern, and the use of common lands in the two villages. In Echalar, the siblings used to compete for the honour of being the chosen heir. However, as farming becomes less desirable, the pressures of competition drive away the children, and they do not send earnings home to maintain the homestead. In Murelaga where the heir is known from birth, there is no sibling rivalry, the other children return 'home' regularly, and send money to keep the place going.

Hansen (1977) points out that Catalonian agriculture was more productive than that of Andalusia because Catalonia had a single-heir system so farm land was not fragmented. In Catalonia, the *hereu-pubilla* system meant that one child in a family inherited the property. Usually this was the first-born son (*el hereu*) but if there were no sons, then the first-born daughter (*la pubilla*) was the heir. This heir got a formal contract when he or she married, specifying that he or she *was* the heir, and what the property consisted of. The other children got a small inheritance, usually in cash. By the time Hansen's research was under way (the 1970s) the *hereu-pubilla* system was in decline, due partly to the tensions in the system (the chosen heir has to be subservient to the father long after most adults would be financially and emotionally autonomous) and partly to the increased legal challenges to the distribution by the heirs' siblings who went to court. One man stuck as the *hereu* told Hansen: 'I only have ten years of life left that I could enjoy, and that guy [his father] is still as strong as an oak' (1977: 101).

By the 1960s, Catalonia was becoming increasingly industrial rather than agricultural, and the inheritance system was increasingly irrelevant as farming became a less desirable source of income. In its traditional form, however, the single-heir system allowed wealth to accumulate and encouraged investment in farm land.

Susan Rogers (1991) reports a similar pattern in France. In 1975 Rogers started research in Ste Foy, a village in the Aveyron, in southern France, a village that was still populated and thriving, amid many severely depopulated areas: 'Ste Foyans proudly refer to their community as one that is 'holding on' (*qui se tient*)' (1991: xi). Rogers suggests that Ste Foy is holding on partly because there is a steady demand for ewe's milk from the village herds from a modern factory which makes Roquefort cheese, partly because there is a strict single-heir system ensuring that each *ostal* (farm/ household/animals and land) passes undivided through the generations, and partly because the farmhouses have been modernised so that young women *are* prepared to marry the heir in Ste Foy. Rogers was told that an *ostal* went either to the eldest son (*l'âineé*), or the son who stays to look after his elderly parents. A daughter can be the heir if there is no son, although Ste Foyans believe a son is the preferred *âiné*.

The classic account of the single-heir system is the work of Arensberg (1937) and Arensberg and Kimball (1940). When they studied rural Ireland the pattern was for all the sons to wait until their father was ready to choose an heir and retire. That son then married, the others had to stay bachelors, leave, or marry a female heiress to another farm. The old couple moved to the end of the house, and were supported till they died, while the chosen heir became the boss. Scheper-Hughes (1979: 41) summarises:

> Arensberg and Kimball's vivid description of a lively farm family life in which patriarchal father delayed retirement and set son against son in the spirited competition for the 'old fellow's' favour and eventual birthright of the farm.

As in Echalar (Douglass, 1975), today the farm is not a prized inheritance. At the time Scheper-Hughes did her fieldwork:

> For at least three decades the selection of an heir for the land [had] been governed by the process of elimination rather than by choice. That is, the last one to escape (usually the youngest son) gets stuck by default with an unproductive farm and saddled with a lifestyle of almost certain celibacy and services to the 'old people'.
>
> (1979: 41–42)

In rural Ireland, as in Echalar, young women do not want to be farmers or even live on farms. Scheper-Hughes studied a village she called Ballybran. There were sixty-four bachelors aged 35 and over and only twenty-seven unmarried women over 35 (nine spinsters and eighteen widows). In the age range of 21–35 there were thirty-five bachelors and only five women:

> the vivacious and mobile young women migrate. They leave behind a large proportion of their beaux who are committed – as the girls are not – to carrying on the family farm and name, a task rendered more absurd each year as these men come to realise that they are not likely to produce any heirs of their own.
>
> (1979: 38)

The reluctance of young women to stay on farms is discussed in more detail in Chapter 5. Germany also has the single-heir system, so in the two German villages studied by Golde (1975: 52)

> it is customary for the parents of a son or daughter, to whom the parents transfer possession of the family farm (usually coincidental with marriage) to stay on in the same house and eat at the same table . . .
>
> The provisions of impartible inheritance allow only one of the heirs . . . to bring in a partner and raise a family in the native household: any siblings who decide to stay in the house . . . may do so only as long as they remain single.

Southern Europe had land endlessly fragmented by inheritance and reunited by marriage, northern Europe land kept intact by a single-heir system. In the south a family with several children could leave them all inheriting too little ground to live off; in the north only the heir could marry and stay at home. Both systems encouraged emigration: of those who did not inherit enough land to feed their families, or of those who were not the heir.

Land ownership and land use are not necessarily the same. There may be landowners who are not present in the community at all, or who only visit for short periods, while the land is worked by tenants or sharecroppers. There may be families who live in the community and farm their own land but own more land than they can work themselves, who hire extra labour, or rent some land to tenants, or have bits of it sharecropped. Then there may be people who are self-sufficient, in that they have enough land to live on (and off) but none to spare. Worse off are people who have to rent land, or sharecrop it, and poorest those who work only as day-labourers, hired by others. Within the farmland of one community all these land ownership and labour patterns may be intermingled. The example here is Cutileiro's (1971) study of a village in the south-east of Portugal near the Spanish border. Vila Velha was surrounded by the mild lands (*terras mansas*) which are flat and good for farming, and the harsh lands (*terra asperas*) which are too hilly for crops. Many of the crops in Vila Velha had been grown since the Roman occupation, especially grain and olives. A few wealthy landowners do not work on the land they own, the majority of the population own and rent enough land to support themselves, while the poorest families are sharecroppers and/or labourers for others. Typically people had several sources of income, so that the café owner also owned some land, and a landowner also ran the village taxi, and so on. In Vila Velha there were 480 landholders still resident, of which twenty-six had enough land to support them and they owned 21 per cent of all the land. The rest have to supplement the produce from their own land with work for others.

The stratification system of Vila Velha was as follows. At the top were the gentry – the *latifundists* – who owned land but did not work it themselves. Many of them did not live in the community at all, but in Lisbon or a provincial city. They were so wealthy that their land was managed for them by a foreman, they were educated and had connections to national life. The equivalent group in Barrett's (1974) village Benabarre are called *Los Señoritos*.

Below the *latifundists* come the *proprietarios*, those who live on their land and farm it with their own family labour. Then come the *seareiros*, or sharecroppers, who farm someone else's land and share the crop with the landlord. In the Vila Velha the landlord got between one-fifth and one-quarter of the crop while the share-cropper kept the rest. Below sharecroppers came the *trabalhadores* (labourers) who were employed by the year, the season, the week or even the day. This is the hardest and most insecure kind of work, and meant no pay when the weather is bad. Cutileiro argued that the older men had a grudging pride in their hard work, while younger men saw no merits in the work and left the village.

There are long debates in literature on peasants and their land and labour (Franklin, 1969; Bailey, 1971b; Rogers, 1987; Holmes, 1989; Galt, 1991). Some researchers have concluded that peasants admire town-based, office-based, white-collar work and regard their own way of life with loathing. Other scholars stress how peasants feel that farm work is the only 'real' work for 'real' men. Peasant farming can be hard, but it is seasonal – so that at a busy time such as harvesting, work can last from dawn to dusk while in slack periods there may only be a couple of hours work to do.

White (1980) argues that in the two central Italian towns she studied the peasants' attitudes to their land and labouring were very different. In the town with a few large landowners and a mass of poor peasants, farm work was despised. In the other town, where there were no large landowners and land tenure was equal and democratic, there was dignity of labour. Agricultural work was a source of pride. This research is described in more detail in Chapter 7.

To a reader used to large, flat green fields, the available land in many Mediterranean countries looks too small in area to grow enough to feed anyone. Jenkins's (1979) study of Alto waxes lyrical about the merits of terracing a hillside to grow crops, but cannot disguise the hard work that farming on such terraces, without any machinery, involves. Connell (1980) gives an idea of a traditional farming economy, based on a study of the Greek islands of Amorgos, Donoussa, Schinoussa and Irakleia. Amorgos did not have electricity in the 1970s, so farming and domestic work were still done by hand or animal power. Connell spent nearly a year on Amorgos studying a way of life that he believed to be dying. The main crops on Amorgos are:

> oats, corn, chickpeas and lentils. Because of the hilly terrain of the islands, most of the crops are cultivated on small strips of land terraced by stone dykes built generations ago to prevent the

erosion of the scanty soil. In many parts the soil is so stony that scarcely anything can be grown but nevertheless the areas are still planted . . . Each family produces its own vegetables – potatoes, cabbages, cauliflowers, french beans, broad beans, artichokes, onions, garlic and lettuce. Summer crops are tomatoes, cucumber, squash, aubergines, peppers and ladies fingers.

(Connell, 1980: 18)

In the early autumn the wild greens (*horta*) appear after the dry summer, and are eaten through the winter. The water supply was limited and most work was done by hand because no-one could use machinery on terraces in stony soil. People grew vegetables for their own use, and kept a donkey, mule, cow or ox to plough with, and kept goats or sheep for milk and fleeces. Connell emphasises the sheer physical labour needed to farm on Amorgos. He went out to help bring in the olive crop. This was done in two ways. Either people spread sheets on the ground under the trees and then, using long sticks beat the branches so the ripe fruit fell off onto the sheets, or they went up ladders and picked olives by hand into baskets. Both are exhausting. Connell worked for six hours, and found that he had only managed to fill two baskets (3.75 kilos) with olives. The locals, who were much more skilled, picked more. Two people working from dawn to dusk can gather 100 kilos, which is a load for two donkeys to carry home at the end of the day.

Calabresi (1987) is a detailed account of the grape harvest (*vendemmia*) in Tuscany, and also describes the wine making and the family diet as it changes over the annual cycle of crops. The wine harvest was too big for the old couple left on the farm to manage without their sons, who had town jobs, but returned to get the grapes in. A mixed team of five adults and several children worked extremely hard for a whole weekend to get in the grapes to make wine for the family for the forthcoming year.

In all the studies of peasant farming those researchers who actually tried it for themselves report on the physical demands of such labour. It is seasonal, and there are quiet periods when little can be done, but at harvest times long hours of back-breaking, sweaty, dirty work are required.

The final theme of this chapter is the division of labour by sex. In many farming cultures there is a clear line between what jobs men can do and what women can do. In the northern Portuguese village studied by Pina-Cabral (1986: 83-84) women were forbidden to climb trees or prune vines (important activities when the village produces *vinho verte* where the vines are trained up into trees).

There is also a feature of farming in Pisticci (Davis, 1973), and other southern European agro-towns, which is the differences between men and women in their use of the land. Pisticci consisted of the town itself and the surrounding agricultural land owned by people who lived there. The whole area was 23,054 hectares, of which the town occupied 25 hectares and the remaining 23,029 hectares were the farm land. Women and children, especially the girls, live most of their lives in the 25 hectares, while men roam the whole 23,054 hectares. In Pisticci, farm work is dishonourable for women, so when extra labour was needed for getting the tobacco crop harvested, Pisticcians paid whole families to come out from the city of Lecce. Lecce women *did* do farm work, and were therefore regarded by Pisticcians as immoral.

Whether or not women were expected to do the same tasks as men, or had different ones, in most peasant cultures a household only survived if both sexes were hardworking. If the woman's tasks were the kitchen garden, the pig and the hens, and the care of the young lambs, plus fieldwork at harvest time, while the man dealt with the grain and the mature animals at pasture, the family only ate if both partners did their share properly. Women were not housewives and mothers, they were workers on the peasant holding. All over Europe the traditional farming systems are collapsing because women no longer want to do 'their' tasks, and young men prefer wage labour to peasant farming.

SUGGESTED READING/ACTIVITY

Robin Jenkins (1979) *The Road to Alto* is an accessible plea for the preservation of peasant farming by a Marxist 'green'.

Chapter 4

The trampled garden
Invasion, refugees, migrants and tourists

They will trample our gardens to mire
They will bury our city in fire

Our women await their desire,
Our children the clang of the chain . . .

(Flecker, 1947: 77)

INTRODUCTION

The theme of this chapter is the movement of populations. The
EEC has seen waves of refugees, fleeing from invasions or persecution; it encourages the ebb and flow of migrant workers seeking
work when it is available and returning 'home' when it is not; and
then there are the tourists, moving around in their millions. This
chapter looks at the lasting impact of the Balkan conflicts of
1912–20 which led to the Greek diaspora of 1922 and its more
recent equivalents in Cyprus and 'Yugoslavia'. The end of colonialism produced populations of returners to France and Portugal
who changed their home countries by their return. Then there is
a body of research on migrants, both temporary and permanent,
and on those who return. Finally, the tourist, a modern form of
population movement, is the newest subject of anthropological
research.

This book is being written as Yugoslavia burns and several
million people are becoming refugees, exiles and forced migrants.
This chapter deals with those who have fled from war, persecution
and 'ethnic cleansing', as well as those who have emigrated in
search of work and those who have returned to their 'homelands'.

REFUGEES AND EXILES

The two most poignant studies of refugees are both about Greeks, by Hirschon (1989) and Loizos (1981). Hirschon studied those Greeks who were forcibly returned from modern Turkey in 1922 (after the war between Turkey and Greece there was an 'exchange' of populations) and settled in distinct neighbourhoods in Piraeus, the port of Athens. Loizos followed the people of his father's natal village into their exile in western Cyprus after the Turkish invasion of the north of the island in 1974. Hirschon's is one of several books on a community where 1922 refugees were settled. There is also Salamone's (1986) account of the 1922 refugees who settled on an island near Mount Athos. Danforth (1989) studied Ayia Eleni, a village of 700 people in eastern Macedonia. In 1976 there were still separate neighbourhoods for the Kostilides, who were refugees in 1922 from Kosti in Thrace who are famous for the *Anastenaria* – a fire-walking ceremony in honour of several Greek Orthodox saints. In 1976 they were still called 'refugees' by everyone else. Then there were villagers who had arrived from Turkey in 1922, and the rest were the 'locals' who had worked for the landowners in the area (who were Turks) before they had to leave in 1922 when the Turks were expelled. Thus fifty years after 1922 the impact of the population shifts was still felt strongly. Cowan's (1990) research site in northern Greece, Sohos, was also used for refugee settlement in 1922, as was Rethemnos on Crete where Herzfeld (1991) has done his most recent fieldwork. Thus we have five ethnographies of contemporary Greece done in the post-1970 period all of which show that the identity of 'refugee' has not faded in fifty years. Greek Orthodox believers are currently coming 'home' from the former USSR, arriving in a Greece they have never seen (Hudson, 1992), and presumably in 2050 their descendants will stand out from those who lived in Greece earlier than the 1990s. Hudson says 50,000 migrants from the former USSR have already moved to Greece, mostly to the northern area of Thrace, where they are displacing the long-settled Muslim population. Hudson sees new housing going up round towns such as Komotini which will 'rapidly transform the religious and ethnic balance of the area'.

The Greeks and the Greek Cypriots are the best-documented groups of refugees, but are by no means the only such populations. Europe since 1900 has seen many such displacements. Jews had to flee Russia and Eastern Europe, and then Nazi Germany. The Spanish Civil War of the late 1930s drove Spaniards into exile, the 1939–45 war displaced millions, as did the division of Europe by the 'iron curtain' after 1945. The German village, Burgbach, studied by Spindler (1973) was settled by an influx of refugees in 1945. In 1935 the village had 1,600 people all of whom were Schwabisch-speaking and Protestant. The American occupying forces settled 450 refugees there, who were from East Germany, the Sudetenland and Poland. These refugees were German speakers not Schwabisch-speaking, Catholic not Protestant, and were not farmers but town-dwellers. By 1950 Burgbach had a population of 2,537. Twenty years later the divisions between old residents and refugees were still visible in the village.

Nor did 1945 see the end of refugees in Europe. The Greek Civil War of 1944–48 produced an exodus of communist Greeks to Albania and Yugoslavia including 30,000 children, and 700,000 Greeks had been displaced (Boatswain and Nicolson, 1989). Next, the Hungarian rising of 1956 produced refugees, as did the Czech one of 1968. The surveys of mother tongues spoken in London (Rosen and Burgess, 1980) and in England (Linguistic Minorities Project, 1985) show traces of these refugee populations in the UK, and similar surveys would reveal an equally diverse spread of refugees in other cosmopolitan cities such as Paris. Another sign of refugees is the restaurant trade: a glance at the range of restaurants available in London can show the refugee pattern; there were no Vietnamese restaurants until the boat people, no Lebanese before the civil war in the Lebanon, and the displaced Croats and Bosnians will produce a new set of Croatian and Bosnian restaurants all over northern Europe. A third sign of refugees is new places of worship: it was Russian refugees who needed the Russian Orthodox cathedral in Knightsbridge, Ukrainian refugees needed Ukrainian Orthodox churches, and so on.

The Greek refugees: a case study

The refugees from the Greek catastrophe of 1922 are a good case study because there is anthropological work on the survivors, and so they may serve as the ethnographic example. The Greek catastrophe – the *diogmos* or 'casting out' – followed the Balkan wars of 1910–22. (The 1914–18 war started earlier and lasted longer in the Balkans.) In 1910 there were about 1.5 million 'Greeks' living in what is now Turkey, at that time the Ottoman Empire in the last years of its long existence. A Greek army invaded the Turkish coast in 1922 and was beaten by Kemal Ataturk. In the aftermath of this defeat half a million Greeks died, and the million who escaped death were evacuated, or fled/escaped to Greece. About 350,000 Muslims were despatched the other way and there are still deserted 'Turkish' villages to be seen in Greece. The Greek army were evacuated through the city of Smyrna (modern Izmir) which had a large Greek community, many of whom died in fires, and the systematic massacre carried out by the advancing Turkish army.

Greece had to cope with a million refugees, who shared a religion and a language, but had little else in common with the Greeks living in Greece. The research done by Hirschon (1989) on those who settled in the neighbourhood of Yerania, in Piraeus (the port of Athens) and still live there today and Salamone's (1986) on those who settled in Ammouliani on the tiny islands under the shadow of the peninsula of Mount Athos show common features. The refugees were and *are* convinced that their lost way of life was more cultured, richer, more truly Greek, and more civilised than that of the 'peasants' inhabiting Greece in 1922. Those who had lived in Smyrna and Constantinople saw their enforced move as a change from a civilised life in great cities to an existence in a scruffy provincial town or a backwater of 'bumpkins'. Although they were penniless refugees they saw themselves as the truly Hellene heirs of Pericles and Plato, the 'real' upholders of Greek civilisation. Herzfeld (1982) is an examination of that Hellene identity in modern Greece although written in a dense and diffi-cult style which cannot be recommended to novice anthro-pologists. The discussion of 'Romaioi' versus 'Hellene' in Fermor (1966) is a more accessible introduction to contemporary Greek ideas of identity.

Hirschon's work shows that the refugee residents of the suburb had remained aloof from other Greeks in Athens, but that the older generation believed that this distinctiveness was dying because it was based on an event fifty years before. A women in her 70s expressed it thus:

> Our 'refugeeness' is disappearing, the old people are dying and whatever one might describe, it is only like a small patch of cloth. We experienced it, but it's like a fairy story to our children.
>
> (Hirschon, 1989: 248)

In Crete, Turks left the town of Rethemnos, and refugees arrived there. Herzfeld (1991: 20) estimates that 3,000 Turks were forced to leave the town, to be replaced by 1,350 refugees. Both groups were exiled:

> The departing Muslims regarded Crete as their home. Their language, for the most part, was Greek. Their departure was as bitter an exile as the reverse flow of Christians, some of them Turkish-speaking, into the Greek territories.

The Cretans already settled in Rethemnos were not welcoming to the refugees:

> For the refugees, though suddenly destitute, were more cosmopolitan than the indigenous Cretan population especially the villagers recently arrived in town . . . Intense mutual dislike resulted. The refugees lamented a fate that placed them among rude peasants while the rural Cretans called the refugees 'Turks' – a clear acknowledgement that in some ways the newcomers were more alien than the *Taurkokritiki* who had departed.
>
> (Herzfeld, 1991: 64)

Herzfeld says 'refugee' was still a children's insult in Rethemnos in the 1970s.

There were no anthropologists travelling with the refugees of 1922 or living alongside them in the immediate aftermath of that diaspora. Loizos's (1981) study of his Greek Cypriot family and friends, displaced from Argaki when the Turks invaded Cyprus in 1974, is as close as we are likely to get to understanding the feelings of such exiles. Loizos describes how the exiles are bereaved, like people whose parents have died, and grieve for their lost land, their houses and gardens and, in important ways, for their identity. One of his friends told Loizos that he expected the partition of Cyprus to be temporary, and that he expected to be able to go home again. Loizos writes, sadly:

> I found it hard to say to him that after many wars the refugees had not gone home, and that partition had become a commonplace 'solution' to both superpower and regional conflicts. Poland, Ireland, Germany, Korea, Vietnam, were all testaments to this. I was sad for him, for his innocence and hope.
>
> (Loizos, 1981: 187)

Exiles

Before leaving this case study of refugees, who in the Greek and Cypriot cases at least fled in family groups, it is important to remember that some individuals have to become exiles alone. Several regimes have dealt with dissidents by confining them to remote regions. Kenna (1991b) is an account of exiles sent to Nisos (a very remote island in the Aegean) during the Metaxas regime (1936–41). The most famous example of such an exile is Carlo Levi, author of *Christ Stopped at Eboli* (1982). Levi was a doctor of left-wing views exiled by Mussolini from Florence to the deep south of Italy in the 1930s. His description of the poverty, ignorance, ill-health, and neglect by Church and state that he found there makes a most poignant account of southern Italy.

A third type of refugee or exile is the returner from the 'lost' colony. Since 1945 Belgium, France, Great Britain, The Netherlands and Portugal have all been driven out of, or voluntarily relinquished, colonial territories overseas. When the ex-colony has gained independence, a number of colonists and expatriates has returned home. After the independence of Algeria in 1962 thousands of *pieds noirs* came 'home' to a France that their families had left sometimes a century earlier. The most recent set of returners are those who came back from the African colonies to Portugal after 1974 (see Goldey, 1983a). Gregory and Cazorla Perez (1985) studied some of the Portuguese who returned from Angola and Mozambique. There were 20,131 such refugees on the Algarve in 1976. Those with education and family connections were settling into the life of the small towns, but those without families sank into poverty.

The feelings of loss reported from studies of refugees can be experienced by those who lose their homes in 'natural' catastrophes such as earthquakes, floods, volcanic eruptions and so on. Those displaced may feel themselves to be exiles, those left behind may feel abandoned.

When Belmonte revisited Naples in the 1980s he found the inner city changed, because of the earthquake of 1980.

> Approximately a third of the local population had been displaced to trailer camps [caravan parks] and second class hotels near the stadium to await the construction of large public housing projects on the periphery of the city.
>
> (1989: 157)

Leah, a prostitute, had loved Naples as it was. She exclaimed:

> It is vanished, Tommaso. It will never revive. My Napoli – there was
> a culture here, no? *Una cultura popolare?* . . . A culture that had
> endured for centuries is destroyed now forever. *Finito! Morto!*
>
> (p. 157)

Although many millions of people have been refugees in twentieth-
century Europe, the numbers of people moving voluntarily in search
of work since 1950 have been much greater. There is no way of
producing a precise count of all those who have migrated in search of
work, because many have done so 'illegally', without the paperwork
that is theoretically necessary. The next section of this chapter deals
with the research on voluntary migration.

VOLUNTARY MIGRATION

There are three types of migration to be covered in this section:

1 migration within one country such as movement from a village
   to a city or from an agricultural area to a tourist coast;
2 migration from one country in Europe to another in search of
   work, such as a Portuguese woman moving to France to work;
3 return migration; such as the same Portuguese woman going
   'home' again.

Internal migration

One of the most interesting accounts of an internal migrant is
strictly outside the scope of this volume, being set in Morocco.
However, the same factors which underlie the hero's migration
within Morocco also propel Moroccans to France and Belgium, so
it illustrates the general themes.

John Waterbury's (1972) *North for the Trade* is the life story of a
Moroccan man, Hadj Brahim, who was living in Casablanca when
he talked to Waterbury. Hadj Brahim was born in the Souss, a
barren dry region in the south of Morocco. The area is so poor
that, Hadj Brahim explained, men had been leaving in search of
work for at least a century. He had left his village in a poor valley
of southern Morocco aged 9, and moved to Casablanca helping a
spice merchant, also from the Souss. By the age of 17 he was
co-manager of a shop, like many other Soussi, who dominated the

grocery trade in the urban north of Morocco. The pattern was to send all the earnings back to the village; the Soussi motto was 'Big spender in the valley, miser in the city.' Men took it in turns to work away, so that there were enough left to protect the respectability of the community's womenfolk, who stayed behind. Before 1945 the customers were mainly the European colonial settlers, but after 1945 Moroccan customers were welcome too. Hadj Brahim felt he had been forced to leave the Souss by poverty, and explained that the Moroccans who chose to go to France, Belgium and elsewhere in the EEC to work in the 1960s were doing the 'same' as he had done, only the journey was longer.

Hadj Brahim's story is a 'success': that is, he moved to better himself and did so. In his account of Soussis' migrations he described two common types of internal migration. First there is seasonal or temporary migration, where a man's permanent home does not change, but work takes him away for periods. Hadj Brahim himself began doing that, but later moved his wife to Casablanca and so became the other type of internal migrant: one who has left permanently or semi-permanently and no longer keeps his main home in the country. The same families can be involved in both types, perhaps trying one and then the other.

All over Europe people born in rural areas move to towns and cities, or to tourist resorts, in search of jobs better than agricultural labour and a status higher than 'peasant'. Kenna (1983) studied Greeks leaving a tiny island for Athens, Kenny (1960) Castilians moving from a village to Madrid, Simon (1976) researched a mountain village in Corsica whose young people head for Paris, and Pitkin (1985) is a life history of a family who left a southern Italian agrotown for the outskirts of Rome where there were jobs.

Pitkin (1985) has told the story of the Tassoni family since the turn of the century, having known them since 1951, when he was doing his doctoral fieldwork in Valmonte. The poverty of the family before 1933, when they moved to Valmonte near Rome from Stilo in Calabria, was still vivid in the mind of Guilia Tassoni when Pitkin collected her life story systematically in 1977, when she was 79. Her husband, Giovanni Tassoni, was the son of a landless labourer, who stood in the piazza every day and hoped to be given a day's work. Giovanni followed him. Guila was child-minding at 7, and at 12 was carrying stones on her head for a mason. Stilo promised little work, even for the hardworking, and Giovanni suffered from malaria, still endemic in Calabria in the

1920s. As a young married couple with small children Giovanni and Guila decided in 1933 they had to get away to find work, and moved to Valmonte. Here there were jobs, and the family eventually got land, and were able to build a house on it. The whole book is a story of gradually rising prosperity, due to migration from the south to the more prosperous area round Rome. In Calabria, Sicily and the rest of southern Italy, such labour migration has a long history which can be read about in, for example, Cornelisen (1980) and Douglass (1983, 1984), with the centre and north of the country 'pulling' Italians in search of better jobs. (Italians also left Italy altogether, a longer-range migration discussed in the next section.) Alpine Italy also suffered migration due to poverty, both seasonal and permanent. Hertz (1913/1983) found that as long ago as 1913 the men in the Soana, an Italian Alpine valley where he studied the pilgrimage of St Besse, worked away from the village for half the year, driven by poverty. Men went as far as Paris to work as glaziers in the winter.

Other European countries also had both seasonal and permanent internal migration. In France, the Alpine village studied by Rosenberg (1988) regularly sent people to Marseille in the winter to sell hot chestnuts on the streets or get work as labourers. There are reviews of the rural–urban migration process in Spain (Buechler, 1983); Italy (Douglass, 1983); Yugoslavia (Simic, 1983); Greece (Sutton, 1983); and Portugal (Leeds, 1987). The impact of internal migrants within Spain has been studied by Woolard (1989) in Catalonia; by Heiberg (1989) in the Basque country, and in several regions in the collection edited by Aceves and Douglass (1976).

Since the beginning of the century able-bodied men have left villages to seek work elsewhere, it has been less usual for women to do so, and the migration of whole families has been more common since the 1950s. The next section examines migration from one country to another.

Guest workers and emigrants in Europe

Halpern (1987) has written about the *pecabla* tradition in Yugoslavia. Halpern was writing before Yugoslavia was torn apart, but the *pecabla* tradition was Macedonian, and was a male migration pattern from isolated mountain villages. The *pecalba* tradition was functioning before the 1914–18 war, when Macedonia was part of the Ottoman Empire. Christian Macedonian men would go as far as Istanbul in search of work, although some only went as far as Belgrade (eighteen days' ride away). Most men got jobs in the building trades. In 1962 Halpern was told of the tradition of men leaving for work, and contemporary guestworkers in Denmark, Sweden and Germany were described as the heirs to the ancient *pecalba* tradition.

Halpern found that much 'Yugoslavian' emigration was a two-stage process. A peasant first got work in a town in Yugoslavia, and then tried working abroad. People from different regions of Yugoslavia had different destinations. with Croatians preferring Germany and Serbians Austria and France. Prophetically, Halpern pointed out that hostilities between Serbs and Croats were frequently played out in Sweden or Denmark. This work of Halpern's contains most of the themes necessary for understanding guestworkers. Such migrations in search of work are rarely new; usually the poor region or nation has been exporting labour for centuries. Migrants may move in stages, trying a town in their own country, before a move to another nation. Migrants from a particular community or region usually go to work in an area where they will find compatriots, and they go with their 'cultural baggage' of racial, linguistic and religious identity which affects who they can associate with in the destination country.

Guestworkers and immigrants have been studied in two main ways. There are researchers who 'follow' emigrants from their home community to their destinations (such as Gregory, 1976; Cornelison, 1980) and there are studies done of guestworkers and immigrants in their destinations (such as Boisvert, 1987; Goodman, 1987; Sontz, 1987). Scholars usually suggest that migrant workers experience both 'push' factors which cause them to want to leave their home community, and 'pull' factors which attract them to the destination. Belmonte (1989: 147) tells of a young man from Naples, 'Pasquale had "fled" to Germany . . . Pasquale worked in a pizza parlour in Dusseldorf and had made a good adjustment to German life'.

Readers of Belmonte's book know that Pasquale had a strong 'push' factor to leave his family in Naples: he was the family scapegoat whose father tormented him. Leaving for Germany was an escape from a violent and stressful family, plus the poverty of Naples. Rhoades (1978) found that the first man to leave Alcudia de Guadix for Germany went in 1961, because he had incurred a debt he could see no way to pay off. This man slipped away illegally, and found a job 'illegally' in Neuss, West Germany. Once he had made enough money to pay the debt he came home, but then went back and other young men from Alcudia followed him and by 1970, there were 700 Alcudians in Neuss.

Leeds (1987) studied three Portuguese villages to investigate who decided to leave and who to stay. In Santa Vitoria:

> the work cycle in cork and olives was about four months. One man in another village of the same ecozone, when asked what they did the other nine months, said, 'we stood on the street corners and starved'.
>
> (p. 35)

Given such comments, Leeds did not find decisions to seek work in France at all surprising. Similar points are made by Mendonsa (1982), Brettell (1986) and Goldey (1983a).

Researchers on Spanish emigration have produced similar arguments. Gregory (1976) studied migrants from an area near Seville, who had gone to Germany because of the lack of work. That is, they were the poorest people, and Gregory found that the conservative middle class tried to prevent their poor 'neighbours' from going as migrant workers. Gregory and Cazorla Perez (1985) is a contrast of government policies about emigration in Spain and Portugal, and it is clear that in the same period the middle classes in the agrotown Gregory studied were discouraging workers from leaving, it was government policy to encourage unemployed Spanish men to take jobs in France and Germany.

There have been many studies of the lives of guestworkers and immigrants in the destination countries. Watson (1977) is a collection on Britain; Gerholm and Lithman (1988) on Islamic guestworkers in western Europe; other works in this area include Rogers (1985), Wilpert (1988a), Liebkind (1989) and Rex, Joly and Wilpert (1988). As many of the immigrants and guestworkers settled in towns and cities, some of the work is covered in Chapter 6. Much of the focus has been on how guestworkers keep their language, culture and identity alive in an alien land. Boisvert (1987) has studied Portuguese families in France, and Giles (1991) is an account of women in a Portuguese neighbourhood in London in 1982-84 and 1989. The neighbourhood had a community centre (*Centro 25 do Abril*), a cafe and shops where Portuguese food and drink were available.

The biggest issue facing guestworkers and immigrants is whether to stay permanently or to go home. For some, there is no chance to stay because the destination country does not allow it; but if the possibility of changing nationality arises, it poses major problems. The Spaniards in Switzerland studied by Buechler (1987) were all facing such dilemmas as to whether to send their children home to Spain and stay themselves, or try to keep their children with them. A man alone can save more money than a whole family; a family abroad produces identity crises especially for the children (Wilpert, 1988b). When the economy of France or Germany takes a recessionary turn more guestworkers leave, when there is an upswing more arrive. The issues surrounding return migrants are the subject of the next section.

Return migration

Robert Rhoades (1979b) was one of the first anthropologists to call for detailed attention to return migration, based on his own study of Alcudia de Guadix near Grenada – the town which provided the setting for the novel *The Three-Cornered Hat*. Anthropologists had neglected to study return migration, and Rhoades set out to remedy that lack by editing a collection of papers on the topic which included his own work on return migrants to Alcudia. The main effect of returners to Alcudia was on the housing conditions. In the 1950s many Alcudians still lived in caves, which were picturesque but rather insanitary. Returners built houses, so the caves were abandoned. Returners did not want to go back to being day-labourers on farms, but tried to buy land or set up small businesses. These are fairly common findings. Subsequently the collection edited by King (1986) has appeared. He says that: 'Return migration has always been one of the more shadowy features of the migration process, principally because of the difficulty of obtaining satisfactory data for this process' (p. 1).

King's own work has been predominantly on southern Italy. King, Strachan and Mortimer (1986) is one account of guestworkers' return to the *mezzogiorno*. The team chose seven communes in Puglia, Basilicata and Calabria where between 1982 and 1983 they conducted 705 interviews with adults who had spent at least a year overseas and had been back for at least one year in the previous decade. The 705 interviewees were members of 486 households. Most of the respondents had been in Germany (40 per cent) or Switzerland (23 per cent), while a few had been in France, Belgium, the USA, Canada and Venezuela. The typical pattern was for a migrant to leave when between 17 and 29 years of age (63 per cent of the respondents) and stay away for an average of nine years mostly in one country. Over half of the migrants had gone alone, even if they were married at the time. The average age on return was 35 years and 84 per cent were home by the age of 54.

King and his assistants asked these returners why they had left, and why they had come back again. Two-thirds of the respondents told the researchers they had left for economic reasons, and most of the rest said they had accompanied the breadwinner (as wives or children) in his search for work. The reasons given for return were not primarily economic. Only 13 per cent of the interviewees gave economic reasons for return, while two-thirds offered 'family' and 'nostalgia' reasons. People said they had returned to find an Italian spouse, to get their children educated in Italy and to look after aged parents. Overwhelmingly, the respondents felt that their period outside Italy had been a success, and most (58 per cent) said they would advise others to try emigration. Only 14 per cent: 'doubted whether the sacrifices of emigration (separation from family and friends, isolation in an alien culture, hard work, etc.) were really worth the rewards' (King *et al.*, 1986: 65).

Bernard and Ashton-Vouyoucalos (1976) collected life histories from fifteen migrant families who had returned to Greece from West Germany and settled in the Athens area. These adults were working class and only three had completed secondary school. The authors comment that these informants were ambivalent about their experience in Germany and their return. Germany was seen as a more efficient society where hospitals were clean and orderly and patients treated with dignity and given the best treatment even when they did not bribe the doctor, but also a place where Greeks were despised as second-class guestworkers. Wages were better in Germany but housing was difficult for Greeks, because of landlords' prejudices. As one woman explained: 'They didn't give good houses to foreigners. They thought us uncultivated and likely to damage the property' (1976: 45). The returners found Greece dirty and unhygienic compared to Germany, but were distrustful of German schooling for their children. While back in Greece they felt 'home' again, but could also see many benefits to life in Germany.

King (1979: 17) set out the argument that the:

notion of the returnee as a bearer of new skills, new ideas and investment capital, eager and willing to help in the development of his country of origin, is by and large, falsely utopian.

King points out that working overseas does not convert a rural labourer into a skilled worker needed in their homeland. Many of the migrant workers take unskilled jobs in their destinations so do not learn any new skills. Those who do gain a skill have been trained to do a particular job for a particular employer, which does not necessarily transfer to an industry at home. Returners are not necessarily wanted by employers in their home countries, because they have been used to higher wages, better conditions and the protection of a trade union, unlike workers who have never left. Most returners seem to want to buy land and/or set themselves up in small businesses, such as taxis, lorry driving, cafés, shops and so on. The main thing returners do is build houses.

> In Portugal, possession of a house is regarded as the best invest-
> ment and status symbol a return migrant could possibly have;
> the 'petit bourgeois' suburban-style houses mushrooming in
> the Portuguese countryside are visibly modelled on those con-
> structed by the same migrant bricklayers in urban France.
>
> (Brettell, 1986: 22)

Mendonsa (1982) has done a study of migration from Nazare, a community of about 10,000 people north of Lisbon, which has an extremely high emigration rate. Nazarenos have three migration patterns: seasonal, return and permanent. Seasonal migration is common among fishermen, who work elsewhere in winter and return to Nazare in summer to fish. Migrants go abroad to get money and returners have invested in tourist accommodation, fishing equipment and motorized vans to transport fish. All these investments can both generate income, and give social status in Nazare. Owning a fishing boat is a high-status investment, because the owner is an employer of others. Return migrant women, and the wives of men who had been away alone, were more likely to be involved in paid work than women who had never been away.

Kenna's (1990 and 1992) two periods of fieldwork on Nisos, a remote Aegean island, in 1967 and 1987, revealed the initial impact of emigration (in 1966–67 many of the islanders were living in Athens) and return (after electricity reached Nisos, retired migrants returned and entrepreneurial ones came home to start new businesses). The harbour and jetty had been improved too (in

1984–86) so that a better ferry service could bring tourists to generate income for the new businesses.

Mandel (1990) has studied Turkish guestworkers in Germany and found similar ambivalences to those reported for Greeks. For Muslims, there may be additional tensions about being a guest-worker, with more prejudice to face and a strong feeling that the 'host' community are heathen, immoral, godless sinners. There are about 2 million Turks in Germany, from several different Turkish subcultures, including many Alevi (a minority sect). Mandel describes how the Turks felt tensions in Germany, but equally felt tensions when they returned 'home'. She found that Turks 'at home' often sought out friends from Germany also 'at home', because these friends understood the tensions of being a returnee family.

Lawless (1986) has studied return migration to Algeria from France. Algeria has had a government reinsertion programme, but only a small proportion of returners get jobs through its offices. Most Algerian returners were driven by the lack of promotion prospects in France and missing their relatives. Skilled workers who came 'home' to jobs in state-owned companies such as the steel plant at El Hadjah were given priority in housing and the availability of such housing was a major factor in the decision of such workers to return.

The third type of population movement is that of tourists – the most temporary, but the one that has most effects on the land-scape. This is the focus of the third section.

TOURISM AND TOURISTS

Social scientists have been reluctant to study tourists. Most of the research has been done on the places tourists visit, to study the impact tourism is making upon the social relations and economy of the area. It is hard to imagine being taken seriously as a researcher if one's project involved flying from Luton airport to Benidorm, hanging out in bars and discos, and flying back again after a week. The researcher who does exactly this in Lodge (1991) is a figure of fun. Yet, studies of those packaged holiday makers would be a useful contribution to social science knowledge.

The social science authors on tourism can be divided into two groups, the prosaic and the symbolic. That is, there are writers who report the facts about tourism and those who want to analyse its symbolism. Smith (1989) is an example of a prosaic commentator, MacCannell (1976) and Graburn (1989) are symbolicists. While the literature on tourism as a symbolic act is intellectually fascinating, it is not rehearsed here, in what is essentially a prosaic book.

Smith (1989) has written a useful account of the basic research issues in tourism, and includes a typology of tourisms: because there is not one, but many types. Smith distinguishes between the following: historical/high cultural tourism; ethnic tourism; folklore tourism; environmental tourism; recreational tourism.

Historical and high cultural tourism is focused on museums, art galleries, cathedrals, archaeological sites, theatres and opera houses. So a week in Salzburg to attend the opera festival, in Bayreuth for the *Ring Cycle*, in Paris for the Louvre, in Berlin for the great Egyptian collections, in Chartres for the cathedral, in the Peloponnese for Corinth, Mycenae, Tiryns and Epidauros or in Jordan to see Petra would be high culture or historical tourism. Much of the tourist trade in Europe is of this type, especially in cities. The objects of the tourist's visits are usually set up to receive visitors, and may be designed to cater for them. In European cities such as Berlin, guide books are available in many languages, such as Japanese, because tourists from these countries are expected.

Ethnic tourism is a term Smith uses to cover trips to see 'really primitive' people in their native habitats: for example, a trip to see Iban in their long huts or Inuit in their igloos.

Folklore tourism is trips to see peasant lifestyles, such as the day trips from the Spanish coastal resorts to see 'typical' villages. The examples of Tajos and Fuenterrabia which follow are of this type.

Environmental tourism is motivated by a desire to see 'natural' features, such as the Grand Canyon in the USA. In Europe this would include visiting the Scottish Highlands, going to Corsica to canoe in mountain streams, mountaineering, windsurfing or surfing in the Atlantic, and going up to the Arctic circle to see the Northern Lights. Here the attraction is not so much people or facilities as geographical phenomena.

Recreational tourism is the most popular, and attracts mass participation. The attractions are the five Ss – either Sand, Sea, Sun and Sex or Snow, Sun and Sex. The idea is to relax with good food, alcohol, good mixed company and some limited physical activity not easily available at home – such as skiing or swimming in the sea.

Valene Smith has not listed 'sex tourism' as a type, but that, too, deserves research. Her five types are not totally exclusive, of course. On any given day Athens is full of people engaged in high culture tourism and those on a day trip from a Greek beach resort; the Scottish Highlands may have some people wanting an authentic Celtic experience (folklore tourism), some who have come for the scenery (environmental) and others on their way to Orkney for the premiere of the new Maxwell Davies symphony (high culture). Most of the research done on European tourist sites has been carried out in places where either skiing or beach holidays are sold, with a few studies of the places where 'folklore' is the attraction. There are not nearly enough studies of the places to which high culture, and environmental tourists come. Good anthropology could result from observing visitors to the museums of Amsterdam and Vienna, as well as from making that journey from Luton to Benidorm.

Much of the available data on the impact of tourism has been gathered in Spain. Oriol Pi-Sunyer (1977, 1989) has charted the changes to a fishing village he calls 'Cap Lloc' on the Costa Brava in Catalonia. When Pi-Sunyer first knew Cap Lloc it was a fishing village like 'Farol' in Norman Lewis's (1984) *Voices of the Old Sea*. Today the village of 6,000 hosts 70,000 tourists in a typical high season week. Pi-Sunyer spent his childhood holidays in Cap Lloc, and then studied it as an adult including spending a winter working on a fishing boat (1978).

One irony about Cap Lloc, and the other resorts developed in Catalonia (which has 40 per cent of the hotel units and 60 per cent of the camping places in Spain), is that under Franco they were promoted as Spanish not Catalan. The image of Cap Lloc did not focus on *regional* differences and cultures – tourists who come to Cap Lloc have expectations of 'Spanish' (actually Andalusian) culture, e.g. bull fights, flamenco, etc. Tourists have it imported from elsewhere for them. Workers from elsewhere in Spain speak Castilian not Catalan and their failure to teach their children Catalan is resented by locals.

Intellectuals in Barcelona fear that tourism will destroy Catalan nationality and culture. Pi-Sunyer found that the growth of tourism has increased class conflict in Cap Lloc, and destroyed some traditional occupations such as boat building altogether. Dymphna Hermans (1981), who studied Cambrils on the Costa Dorada, argues that the tourist boom there had led to a significant redistribution of wealth. Less-favoured heirs had always inherited land closer to the sea, which was less agriculturally productive.

When tourism came this marginal land was sold for tourist development for a fortune in local terms.

Catalan intellectuals fear that tourism will destoy Catalonian culture, and similar fears about tourism destroying folk culture are expressed by Greenwood (1989) from his study of the town of Fuenterrabia in the Spanish Basque country. This town has the *Alarde*, a public ritual which celebrates victory over a French army in 1638. The French siege was beaten off after sixty-nine days and the town was given certain privileges for its heroism.

The *Alarde* was a community ritual. Fuenterrabia had seven sections, a fisherman's quarter, the old walled citadel and five wards. Each section sent representatives to the procession, including young men with shotguns, a young woman dressed as a water carrier, and children dressed in Basque costume who play drums and Basque flutes. There are also occupational groups in the procession, such as the woodcutters (*hacheros*), and the mayor and town council on horseback. Greenwood claims that the *Alarde* was a procession with bands but was also: 'a statement of collective valour and of the quality of all the people of Fuenterrabia' (Greenwood, 1989: 175). In the 1638 siege everyone stood together – rich and poor, men and women and children, the farmers, the merchants and the fishermen, all the citizens of the wards. Greenwood argues that the *Alarde* was a ritual of solidarity and unity reaffirming local identity, not a show for others. However, it does happen in the summer – when tourists swell the population of the town to four times its normal size.

When Greenwood first studied the *Alarde* in the early 1970s he thought its future was uncertain, because locals no longer wanted to march in it. Greenwood's diagnosis of the trouble was as follows. In 1969 the national Spanish government opened the castle as a *parador* as part of a plan to increase tourist revenue in Fuenterrabia. However, the narrow streets hardly allowed anyone to watch the *Alarde* which had not mattered, because the whole town took part, so there had not been any 'audience'. Responding to the new tourist audience in 1969 the Municipal Government decreed that the *Alarde* should be done twice for the benefit of tourists. Once it had became a performance for tourism local enthusiasm waned and by 1972 there was even talk of paying people to take part.

In 1977 when he first wrote about this Greenwood was angry. He argued that making 'cultural' things part of a tourist package can (and does) ruin them by stripping them of their authenticity. Greenwood argued that tourism accentuates existing social cleavages and may reduce 'local culture' to a 'meaningless performance' which is sold to tourists.

In fact, the *Alarde* became a political event, because it was a *Basque* celebration, and got swept up into the resurgence of Basque nationalism in the late 1970s (see Heiberg, 1989). So Greenwood was still angry but, by 1989, his initial fears that the *Alarde* would become an empty charade had abated somewhat.

Greenwood's general stance is hostile to tourism but other anthropologists have not been so negative. A contrasting view is expressed by Fraser (1973) in his study of Tajos, a village in the hills behind Malaga, as it changed between 1957 and 1970. Tajos became a 'typical' Andalusian village to which outings came from the coastal resorts. This was one of the two ways tourism has altered Tajos. As well as the day-trippers, there were also jobs on the coast. Before tourism, there was only work in Tajos for 30 per cent of the males, the other 70 per cent now get buses to the coast to jobs there every day. For the first time in a century – perhaps the first time *ever* – every able-bodied male has work, and so do many of the young women.

Wages in Tajos have risen and, despite inflation, family incomes have risen too. As an example of growing prosperity in 1957 there were two lorries, two taxis, one scooter, no private cars and no public transport. Mail came to the village by donkey. In 1970 there were twenty lorries, five taxis, ninety private cars, a swarm of scooters, a bus to the nearest town every hour and a bus to Malaga twice daily.

Thus the village was now connected by public transport, and there was lots of private transport too. Tajos people were now mobile, and connected to the rest of Spain. Fraser also commented that Tajos looked different. The houses had been done up, health and hygiene had improved, and the distinguishing marks of class differences in dress had gone. There were new shops and trade in Tajos (i.e. souvenirs). Also, 300 foreigners were living in the Tajos area, in houses built by locals who had developed building trades.

Moore (1976a) charts the impact of tourism on Mallorca. Since 1950 the growth of tourism and the integration of Mallorca into the Spanish and the wider world economy has broken down the ostracism of the Xueta, a previously outcast group (see Chapter 6). The island is 35 miles wide and 75 miles long, yet the airport is the fourth busiest in Europe. The growth of tourism led to the halt of the decline of Palma and of the population generally on the island, plus the immigration of skilled and specialist people. By 1976 half the growing population of Palma was immigrants from other parts of Spain. This in turn has produced new urban patterns for Palma – the shoreline is full of accommodation for tourists, while inland new accommodation for Spanish immigrants is being built.

One of the most positive views of tourism's impact on a rural area comes from Villepontoux's (1981) account of a French village he calls Valloire (confusingly taking the same pseudonym as the Hutsons (1971) did for their village). Villepontoux worked in the Maurienne, a region with a population of 47,000. Most of the villages had an agricultural and pastoral economy. Tourism in the region goes back to 1900 but has grown to be *mass* tourism since 1945. Mass tourism is due to the rise of a large middle class in France and elsewhere in Europe, who can afford holidays. There was industry in the region but it is now in sharp decline. Agriculture in the region is now mainly cash crops (lavender, apples and peaches, grain, lamb) but most farmers are old – and agriculture can no longer compete with the productivity of farming in the lowlands. Tourism is now rivalling industry and agriculture as a major source of employment in Valloire.

Valloire's population has grown since 1950 from 750 to 1,100 in 1978. This is partly due to immigration (23.5 per cent of the 1978 population), mostly French and a few Italians. Villepontoux (1981: 143) outlines the ways in which the French government supports tourism. He points out that government does not interfere with private enterprise, but there are state-organised ski holidays for urban children in children's camps, and adult vacation homes for state employees (*collectivités*). Valloire has two of the latter, one for Renault workers from Le Mans, and a second for civil servants from the Department of Domestic Affairs. Valloire is a popular not a fashionable resort. Tourism has an annual cycle like farming used to have. February is schoolchildren's ski parties, then March is adult skiers, then April is children again. From May to June Valloire is quiet, but in July and August the children's holiday camps open for them to take summer holidays in the mountain air. The village is at its busiest between Bastille Day (14 July) and 15 August (a major celebration in Catholic countries, for it is the day the Virgin Mary went up to Heaven: the Dormition or Assumption), and Valloire is particularly popular when the *Tour de France*

goes through. Villepontoux provides an analysis of all the accommodation, jobs and businesses that have developed in Valloire to
serve tourists, and he is optimistic about its beneficial effects.

This contrasts sharply with other writers on Alpine villages (e.g.
Blaxter, 1971; J. Hutson, 1971; S. Hutson, 1971; Rosenberg, Reiter
and Reiter, 1973; Rosenberg, 1988). John and Susan Hutson did
research in a French Alpine village, which they also called Valloire
(although as far as one can tell it is not the same place). In 1900
the population of their Valloire was around 1,000 but by the early
1950s most villagers had emigrated to Marseille, and it was down to
400. Tourism was seen as the salvation for the village, but the
material collected by Susan and John Hutson shows that tourism
destroys the social fabric. This material is discussed in the next
chapter on peripheral regions.

SUGGESTED READING/ACTIVITY

Peter Loizos's (1981) *The Heart Grown Bitter* is an excellent study of
a refugee group. David Lodge's (1991) *Paradise News* is a good
introduction to the sociology of tourism.

Chapter 5

The smokeless homes
Peripheral regions in western Europe

If there be any grief
It is when pale October
Relentless tree-disrober
Conceals the smokeless homes

(Flecker, 1947: 63)

INTRODUCTION

This chapter deals with the peripheral regions of western Europe, such as the Mediterranean:

> Viewed in terms of relative economic and political power, Europe has a strong centre and a marginal periphery. If its prosperous core lies under the smog of the Ruhr, its under-developed periphery is washed by the Mediterranean.
>
> (Boissevain, n.d.: 13)

Another part of the periphery is the 'Celtic fringe' (see Day and Rees, 1991): Wales, Scotland (especially the Highlands and islands), Ireland, Brittany and Cornwall. Then there is the Atlantic fringe, consisting of Portugal and Galicia. These areas all suffer from being a long way from Brussels, Paris and Frankfurt, but their climates and social systems are very different. Their commonest problem, and the reason they are discussed in one chapter, is that it is those areas which, as Hudson and Lewis (1985: 18) put it, suffer from the loss of population due to migration.

> The selectivity of the out-migration process leads to an increasingly feminized and aged population, a decline in labour input into agriculture and a consequent fall in agricultural output

and income. This, in turn, causes a deterioration in services and living standards, as well as a lack of capital for investment in creating new job opportunities. Although the precise mixture of these (and other) causes of decline have varied from one area to another, the decaying ruins of thousands of villages from Amarante to Anatolia are stark reminders of the human costs of creating the booming cities of the 1960s.

The booming cities are the subject of Chapter 6: this chapter focuses on the peripheral areas. It is important to recognise that decaying villages are not a unique response to the 1960s, for villages fell into decay in medieval Europe (for example, abandoned when plague struck) and were left in the nineteenth century as well. However, the speed of the changes in the rural areas has been striking. Pitt-Rivers (1976: viii) stressed the speed of the changes in Spain between 1950 and 1976:

> the south of Europe . . . has followed a route of transformation which recalls the scenes of social desolation with which the anthropologist was familiar elsewhere: 'ghost' villages whose inhabitants have quit for an economically 'better' life in the city, 'grass-widow' villages whose menfolk are gone to work in the industry of the north of Europe, tourist belts whose inhabitants have sold their unprofitable plots for the construction of villas and motels in which they now make more *money* as seasonal domestic workers than ever they wrung from the soil.

The chapter explains the ideas of centre and periphery, and examines life in the regions characterised by 'smokeless homes'. In a paper on emigration from rural Portugal Anthony Leeds (1987) asked 'What is there to stay for?' and this chapter explores that question. It also deals with gender differences in the flight from rural areas: the issues highlighted for the west of Ireland by Scheper-Hughes (1979). Before dealing with those questions, a brief reprise of the bias in the anthropological work is presented, a case study of one peripheral region (Corsica) is outlined, and the debate about one notorious backward region, the *mezzogiorno* of Italy, is summarised. The chapter ends with case studies of pockets of prosperity in peripheral regions: three exceptions that prove the rule, and a brief discussion of whether tourism can 'save' peripheral areas.

The bias in the fieldwork

Anthropologists of Europe have been much more interested in studying peripheral regions and communities than well-populated and
prosperous areas. As Driessen (1992: 3–4) puts it: 'Anthropologists
seem to have a special predilection for studying marginal phenomena
. . . highly specific miniature settings . . . observation in small, well-
ordered communities'. For example, Anthony Galt (1982) did his
first piece of fieldwork on the tiny island of Pantellaria off the coast of
Sicily. Most Sicilians never visit Pantellaria, and many Italians know
nothing about life there. This research is typical of the material on
Italy as attacked by Crump (1975: 20).

> Too many scholars appear to assume that the canons of *anthro-*
> *pological science* are satisfied by forcing the Italian population
> through a sort of sieve to leave only a residue of relatively
> isolated, partly illiterate, technically retarded, rural com-
> munities, sometimes with a non-Italian local dialect.

Crump's attack on anthropological work on Italy could be equally
levelled at the researchers on Portugal, Spain, France, Greece,
Cyprus, Malta and Ireland. Thus Kenny and Knipmeyer (1983: 38)
on Spain:

> Most anthropologists – foreign and national – concentrated their
> efforts on examining rural life, following the peasant studies tradi-
> tion in the decades of 1950 and 1960 . . . There was little if any
> thought given to studying a town or city on its own merits.

Similarly, Vermuelen on Greece:

> few anthropologists have chosen the city as their major research
> site. This neglect of urban areas by anthropologists thus con-
> firms their well-known preference for the often small and more
> isolated villages of the Mediterranean.
>
> (1983: 109)

The anthropological literature on France is dominated by studies of
rural Brittany, the Alpine villages and Corsica: all peripheral regions.

INTERNAL COLONIALISM AND PERIPHERY THEORY

French intellectuals and regional separatists made the idea of
internal colonialism popular during French decolonisation in the

1950s and 1960s. Contemporary British and Irish debates about internal colonialism and periphery theory stem from Hechter (1975). He is an American who wrote a history of the relationship between England and its three 'internal colonies' of Wales, Scotland and Ireland. The ideas aroused a good deal of contro- versy, especially over the issue of whether Wales, Scotland and Ireland actually shared enough features in their relations with England to be treated as equivalent by Hechter. Evans (1991) is a recent demolition of Hechter's ideas. Briefly Hechter argued that internal colonies get stuck with a particular set of economic and social circumstances because of domination by the core. Hechter saw England as a dominant colonising power, having three types of exploited territories: dependent peripheries, internal colonies and actual colonies. A dependent periphery would be Cornwall, Wales is an internal colony and the Falkland Islands and Gibraltar real colonies. A peripheral region is geographically distant, with- out good transport, and suffers a lack of economic development, but the inhabitants feel they are citizens. An internal colony has many of the features of a periphery, *but* the inhabitants have a separate culture (e.g. a language, a religion, an identity) from the dominant core culture which the dominant core culture deni- grates, despises and tries to suppress. A similar argument could be advanced for France, Spain and Italy.

For the purposes of this chapter the idea of 'internal colonies' is *not* used, and the notion of a peripheral region is deployed in a geographical sense to mean any region suffering because it is distant from the core of the nation, or of the EEC.

Inland Corsica: a peripheral region

Corsica is a typical example of a peripheral region, especially the mountainous interior. Kofman (1985) has charted the decline of Corsica from an autonomous region into a dependency. She com- pares Corsica with the Breton and Occitan regions of France and stresses how the regionalist or nationalist movements in all three adopted the theory of internal colonialism. This had been pro- pounded in France to explain the state of the North African colonies (Algeria, Tunisia and Morocco), and when they were decolonised the theory was applied within France:

> It was argued that these regions were economically exploited and culturally subjugated in the same way as France's overseas

colonies, where the core collectively discriminated against a culturally distinct people.

(1985: 263)

The core in France is the Paris basin and the associated French language, the internal colonies are Brittany, Occitan and Corsica.

The Breton, Occitan and Corsican movements demonstrated not only the effects of past colonialism and policies of national unity, but also the continuing process of economic, social and cultural colonialism carried out by the state and capital.

(Kofman, 1985: 263)

Against this background Kofman explores the changing nature of Corsica, which only became part of France in 1768. (It had been 'owned' by the Italian city of Genoa.) In the 1950s Corsica had a homogeneous population which spoke Corsican, then central government regional development programmes brought outsiders to the island. In 1954 there were only 191,000 Corsicans left on the island which was the poorest region of France. The Paris government had a (1957) plan to make Corsica richer by encouraging tourism and eradicating malaria. In 1962–66 with the 'loss' of Algeria, 15,000 repatriates arrived to settle, mostly on the east coast of the island. Corsica was drawn into the French economy but as a dependency: people lived on their welfare and return migrants' wages. The population was rising so that in 1975 there were 227,425 inhabitants, but farms were still being abandoned. Corsica changed from being a self-sufficient island to a dependency of France. The overview of the changing nature of Corsica can be illustrated in a detailed case study of one village.

Simon (1976) has done a detailed ethnography of one such village in the mountains of the interior he has called Pinnellu which had an official population of 1,023 but actually there were only 180 people living there. The rest of the population were on the electoral roll, but lived and worked on the coast of the island, or on the French mainland. Much of Simon's ethnography centres on the study of the family and how the reputations of men and women are established and maintained. This work will be discussed in more detail in Chapter 9. The distinction in a man's social standing being *furbu* which means crafty and 'street-wise' or *punizutu* which means being slow-witted and 'bumpkin-like' is closely related to the out-migration from the village. Simon traced out-migrants from the village. Many were in French government employment. They will retire back to Corsica but to the coast and only come to the village in summer. Young men who stay in the village are stigmatised as too stupid to get decent jobs, that is, *punizutu* not *furbu*. They are condemned to bachelorhood because women refuse to marry men who are going to stay in the village. Simon's grim account of a dying village, in which the bright young people stay only until they have passed the government exams to enter the postal service, police force or civil service, is reinforced by two French feminist authors.

Quastana and Casanova (1984) offer an explanation for women's disenchantment with 'traditional' rural life in the Corsican mountain interior villages. The coastal towns have always been settled by French and Italians and so have not been purely 'Corsican' for many years. Traditional Corsican society is a male-dominated one. The population lived in male-headed extended families. Women had to be obedient and the honour/shame code (see Chapter 9) was strong. There was a strong division of labour, women's agricultural work was different from men's, and the sexes sat separately in church. Men and women used separate bits of the village. Quastana and Casanova paint a picture of a dour patri-archal family structure in which women were segregated and tightly controlled. Women's only strategy for choosing a less hostile family to marry into was to prefer cousin marriage despite Roman Catholic disapproval of marriage between first cousins – when marrying a male cousin a woman at least 'knew' her husband. Women, especially mothers, have power in the house-hold not in wider society; for a woman to have sons gives her power – she raises them.

Quastana and Casanova contrast that dour past with life in Corsica in the 1980s. Integration of Corsica into the French economy has destroyed the traditional extended family because of the arrival of exiles from Algeria, the rural exodus and the penetration of French values. Today most of the population live on the coast and 'tradition' is a nostalgic memory only for *men*. Old women say that young women are lucky not to have been there when they had to 'slave like beasts'. French penetration is seen as liberating for women by women. So girls leave villages for towns and abandon the Corsican language as a symbol of their 'modernity'. Quastana and Casanova argue that the Corsican free-dom movement is a very *male* movement. They claim women are ambivalent about the nationalist movement as traditional values involved repression of women. McKechnie (1993) and Jaffe (1993) are also ethnographies of Corsica.

In literate societies ideas about the impact of internal colonialism or the consequences of being a peripheral region become part of the discourse of the inhabitants themselves. McKechnie (1993) explores this for Corsica, Schweizer (1988) for Sardinia and McDonald (1986) for Brittany. Schweizer's is a particularly interesting account, by a Swede, of how different ideas about internal colonialism and marginalisation have become part of political debate in Sardinia.

Other peripheral regions

A parallel analysis is Kielstra's (1985) on the rural Languedoc. He argues that until the Napoleonic wars, Languedoc was an important area in Mediterranean trade, but the UK navy's domination of the Mediterranean spoilt it. Then, in the 1930s, cheaper products from Algeria destroyed agricultural prosperity and the de-population of the mountains began. Between 1855–1875 the region was reasonably prosperous, but then in 1876, phylloxera struck. This disease killed the vines which produced the grapes for wine. In the 1890s the vines recovered, but by then cheap Algerian wine had stolen the market. Since 1900 wine growing has only survived due to government policies encouraging and subsidising co-operatives for wine making. Most vineyards are now small and run by men in their 50s and 60s. Agriculture is being abandoned, as young people do not want to farm in the Languedoc. Kielstra uses the concept of 'relictual space' (*zone reliquaire*) to describe the Languedoc.

> Such *relictual spaces* are typically areas where moderately favour-able agricultural conditions led in the pre-industrial period to a relatively dense population of small peasant-owners . . . In the present, however, faced with a highly competitive international market system, the concentration of wholesale activities in the hands of large corporations and high rates of interest on credits, small farmers are no longer able to keep their enter-prises economically viable.
>
> (1985: 247)

In small rural communities, the population is increasingly made up of *bricoleurs* (an untranslatable French word which means doing a bit of this, a bit of that and surviving), who own a bit of land and do a bit of wage-labour and hold a part-time job and draw state benefits.

The inner Mani in Greece is another typical peripheral region. In the 1990s the population is less than half what it was in 1939. Those living elsewhere in Greece return for holidays, the olive harvest and to bury the dead (Seremetakis, 1991). Similar analyses have been provided of rural Evia (du Boulay, 1974), of Echalar in the Basque country (Douglass, 1975) and of Ballybran in the west of Ireland (Scheper-Hughes, 1979).

The peripheral region of Europe which has generated most social science is the southern half of mainland Italy with the islands of Sicily and Sardinia, the *mezzogiorno*. This is the largest region of poverty and underdevelopment in a rich country in Europe. As King summarises it (1984: 180):

> The problem of the backwardness of the South has been the foremost issue of national concern throughout the period since unification. No Italian topic has attracted so much polemic and scholarly debate both within the country and without.

Other writers agree: 'The *mezzogiorno* is stereotypically the most backward and poverty-stricken area of the nation' (Douglass, 1980: 338). Mingione (1985) argues that while southern Italy is the largest backward area in any industrialised country, after thirty years of government policies designed to do something about that underdevelopment, the pattern of wealth and poverty is now complicated. Mingione argued that there are patches in the *mezzogiorno* where the only work is in agriculture and that agriculture is still traditional and backward; patches where agriculture has been modernised and is relatively efficient; and patches where government-owned factories and industrial sites have produced pockets of 'developed' prosperity. Mingione himself surveyed the impact of a petro-chemical plant in Syracuse and other government-sponsored industrial developments in the south. He concludes that the 'black economy', the 'informal sector', becomes a vicious circle that traps people.

Amin (1985) did a parallel study on the impact of Fiat's factories at Bari and on Sicily. By 1970 Fiat had decided not to invest any more in Turin, which had become crowded and expensive and where the labour force was both well-organised and committed to bargaining hard for benefits and wages. There were government grants available for industry prepared to build in the south, so Fiat built new branch factories at Bari on the mainland and in Sicily.

Amin says the popular image is that these branch factories are unprofitable, but she is convinced this is not true, aruging that they are good for Fiat. The labour force is men over 30 who also have some farm land, and are prone to take unauthorised time off from Fiat to farm. However, they do not strike, so the working days lost are, according to Amin, about the same as they would be in Turin. Amin's verdict is that these factories are good for Fiat but do not do much to change the *mezzogiorno*.

These are both studies of pockets of industrial development. The case of Locorontondo, an island of agricultural prosperity in a backward region, is presented in the final section of this chapter. The main focus of this section is the traditional agricultural areas, where poverty, out-migration and 'backwardness' dominate.

There are four main social science explanations for the continuing underdevelopment and poverty of the *mezzogiorno*. All have some plausibility. There are geological and geographical explanations, political ones, economic ones, and social ones. These are briefly explored in turn.

First there are geological and geographical reasons for poor agricultural performance. The soil is thin and stony, the rainfall inadequate, the sand-bearing wind (the *sirocco*) from north Africa maddening, and malaria was still endemic in the 1930s (Levi, 1982; Pitkin, 1985). Overpopulation is also 'blamed' for the poverty of the south: the land cannot support the population.

The political explanations centre on either the theories of patronage (which are explained in Chapter 7) or the ideas about core and periphery set out above. The latter are supported by many instances of money voted in Rome never reaching the projects in the south (Schneider and Schneider, 1976), the former by all the research on patron–client relationships, such as Galt (1974). Patronage and clientelism is a vicious circle, because the more a patron's success and status depend on being able to pull strings for individual clients the less he or she has to gain from efficient government. Thus the most able people have no incentive to 'reform' an inefficient and even corrupt political system. Social scientists who 'blame' the political system of Italy for the poverty of the *mezzogiorno* point out that the state in Rome takes almost all responsibilities away from localities, restrictive laws prevent initiatives and very limited powers exist at local level.

Then there are the economic theories which focus on the problems of land ownership and land tenure. Much of the *mezzogiorno* was owned by absentee landlords, who lived in cities most of the year, leaving bailiffs to run the estates. Wealth was taken from the land, not ploughed back into irrigation schemes, walling fields to keep out goats, planting windbreaks, buying machinery, improving crop strains or training the labour force. Where peasants owned the land, the multiple-heirs system constantly subdivided holdings. Many peasants were forced to sharecrop on an annual basis, which does not promote investment. Schneider and Schneider (1976), for example, blame much of Sicily's poverty on the land tenure system.

Silverman (1968) was quite convinced that the agricultural system, especially the land tenure arrangements, had an important part to play in southern poverty. She produced a detailed comparison between central Italy (Tuscany and Umbria) and the south in terms of how, for a century at least, the organisation of land tenure, the organisation of capital other than land, and the deployment of labour has been different. The farming of central Italy had been productive and had led to modernised agriculture, while that of the south stayed primitive. Silverman's argument is detailed, and has been summarised here. Briefly she argues that in central Italy the farm land was arranged in *farms*, so that all the different kinds of land (arable, olive grove, vineyard, orchard, meadows, pasture, woodland) were together, next to each other, as one parcel of ground. In the south, land is in scattered plots, of irregular sizes, distributed unevenly across the area mixed up with everyone else's plots, so that it cannot be worked rationally. In the central zone the family picking fruit can keep an eye on the grazing sheep, in the south the goat may be tethered 10 miles away from the olive grove.

In central Italy the large landowners grouped their tenant farms into groups of eight to ten farms, so equipment could be pooled, and the farms were let on long tenancies, often lasting over several generations, so that estates did not get broken up. The south had no such groupings, the land division was unstable with constant divisions and reunifications with deaths and marriages. At the heart of Silverman's contrast is the central Italian institution, the *mezzadria* system. This was a contract between landowner and tenant, which was between the families, lasted several generations and provided stability. The tenant family lived in a farm house on the land, and kept half the crop, half the profit from any cash sale and all the produce from their kitchen garden. In the south there was a multiplicity of forms of land tenure. There were absentee landlords, peasant owners of plots, and landless labourers. The same person might own one wheat plot, sharecrop another, rent a bit of pasture, and own one olive grove, moving each week from work on a bit of 'owned' land, a bit of sharecropped land, a bit of rented land and back to another sharecropped patch. All the renting and sharecropping arrangements were *unstable*, lasting only one year at a time with no promises of renewal. The southern farmer did not live on 'his' land, either, but in an agrotown, adding a journey on foot or mule back to and from each bit of ground every time a task needed doing.

Silverman argues that the *mezzadria* contract ensured that both landowner and tenant invested in the land – that is both spent profits on irrigation, drainage, walls, ditches, new trees, machinery, better strains of seed and so on. In the south there is no incentive to invest in land that may go out of the family any moment, so people invest elsewhere, especially in the agrotown.

The roles of the personnel are also different in central and southern Italy. In the *mezzadria* system of central Italy the landowner (*padrone*) lived on or near his estate, not away in a city. In the south the large landowners were uninvolved, and absentees, and lived in Palermo, Naples or even Rome. In central Italy the estates were run for the *padrone* by an agent or factor (*fattore*), who gave technical advice, but the *mezzadro* (the head of the tenant family) and his whole family had their own ties of loyalty to the *padrone*. The whole family was the tenant, and the whole family worked on the farm. In the south the agent was not an agricultural expert, but a rent collector and enforcer, and the cultivators worked as isolated individuals in an uncoordinated way.

Silverman then lists a whole set of consequences that follow from the land tenure systems. The central Italian community form was dispersed countryside settlement with large extended families, a set of neighbourhood work exchange relationships (the *aiutarella*), stable political and class relations, and a rich community life with many organisations. The south had large agrotowns with an empty countryside, small nuclear families, no stable work exchange system, unstable class and political relations dependent on shifting patronage relationships, and weak community organisations. For Silverman, then, the south would have developed into a stable, wealthy region if it had had the *mezzadria* system of land tenure.

The 'social' explanation was controversial when first proposed, and has caused the most anger since. In 1958 an American called Banfield published an attack on the people of Montegrano, an agrotown in the province of Potenza. He stated that the reason Montegrano and other towns and villages like it in the *mezzogiorno* were so underdeveloped and poverty struck was 'amoral familism', which he defined as a strategy to: 'Maximise the material short range advantages of the nuclear family; assume that all others will do likewise' (1958: 83). Banfield felt confident that all the poverty of the *mezzogiorno* was the fault of the peasants themselves: they did not cooperate, save, make long-term plans, collaborate on schemes to better their communities or even use their votes wisely. This attack on Montegrano, and by implication a whole region, was received with anger and scorn by anthropologists. Davis (1977) does not even cite Banfield, but attacks another text as 'the second worst book' on the Mediterranean, making it clear that Banfield's was the worst. Critiques of Banfield can be found from Silverman (1968), Douglass (1980, 1984), Davis (1970), Miller (1974), Schneider and Schneider (1976), Miller and Miller (1978), Berkowitz (1984), Pitkin (1985) and many others. Herzfeld (1987: 35) is particularly scathing, pointing out that if the people of Montegrano preferred family allegiance to bureaucratic values, calling them 'backward' is exactly the kind of value-laden label that powerful anthropologists love to impose on their 'subjects' to reinforce their superiority.

> For Banfield, the definitive failure of the Italian peasants lay in their preference of family allegiance over bureaucratic values. He thus endorsed one of the key assumptions of the nation-state concept, which makes the formal political structure the highest incarnation of national aspirations.
>
> (1987: 12)

Banfield's argument rests on

> the statist view of bureaucracy and civic institutions as above human agency both politically and morally.
>
> (1987: 154)

Herzfeld calls amoral familism part of the

anthropological stereotype of Mediterranean rural people as willing to put personal and family interests over general moral considerations.

(1987: 35)

This, for Herzfeld

is strongly indicative of the imbalance of power between those who confer such stereotypes and those to whom they are applied.

(1987: 35)

As Herzfeld later moves in for the kill:

only a Eurocentric, statist definition of virtue could define family allegiance as 'amoral'.

(1987: 128)

There are two important issues related to Banfield's thesis. We can ask whether his description of Montegrano was accurate and if so, whether it applied to other agrotowns, other areas of the *mezzogiorno*. We can also ask whether his diagnosis of the underdevelopment was correct: that is, had he understood why life was lived as it was?

Many of the commentators have suggested that Banfield's observations were simplistic, but not fundamentally wrong. He did not speak the local dialect, or do prolonged fieldwork, and seems to have missed the cofraternities, festival committees and recreational clubs that exist in all the other agrotowns and so, presumably, did in Montegrano. (Cofraternities are brotherhoods dedicated to a saint, whose members ensure that members are properly buried and masses said for the soul.) Banfield also 'missed' patronage ties, godparents and friendships, all of which are reported from all over southern Italy, so he either studied Montegrano carelessly or it was *much* more anomic than any other community researchers have ever found.

Douglass (1980) is a review of the debates surrounding Banfield's thesis in the first twenty years after its publication. Douglass argues that most scholars do not object to the accuracy of the description of Montegrano but *do* object to the causal chain he set out. For many commentators amoral familism is the *result* of generations of poverty and poor government not the cause. Pitkin (1985: 210), for example, is clear that bad government causes amoral familism, and Berkowitz (1984: 83) that it is not so much that the family is so strong but that everything else is so weak: 'the wider social structure is so atomized and the State so ineffective in performing its ostensible duties'.

The political system is described in Chapter 7 and there is more on family life in Chapter 9. Here it is sufficient to state that other ethnographers are sceptical of Banfield's theory, and either dispute his findings or his causal model.

Whether or not there was ever any 'truth' in Banfield's theory, the poverty of southern Italy was solved by many individuals and families by emigration. Douglass (1980, 1984) studied Agnone, a town with housing for 20,000 that had 4,000 residents in the 1970s. For a month in the summer Agnone was full and bustling, for the rest of the year it was 'dead'. Most of the remaining households were either grandparents and grandchildren while the middle generation were away in the north of Italy or in Germany, or *vedove bianche* (white widows), women whose men were away. The area was never good agriculturally, and when Douglass studied it, the main 'industry' was education, because Agnone had the secondary schools for the region. There were 148 teachers living in Agnone, and teaching jobs were much sought after. The families whose poverty so shocked the Canadian Cornelison (1976), solved their problems in Basilicata by emigrating: to Turin and to Germany. So too did the family studied by Pitkin (1985). For thousands of southerners, the problems of the south are solved by leaving. This 'solution' does ease pressure on the land, but drains the south of the enterprising and talented either permanently, or for their most economically productive years. The mass emigration is one way in which the *mezzogiorno* is a typical peripheral region.

One problem that has not been reported from southern Italy is that of 'bride famine'. In many rural areas of Europe the biggest threat to the survival of communities is the lack of younger women who want to live on farms, work on farms, and be married to farmers.

The bride famine

One of the major problems in peripheral regions is the 'bride famine'. Quastana and Casanova (1984) and Simon (1976) both argue there is a shortage of young women wanting to marry and stay in one peripheral area: inland Corsica. The same pattern is found in western Ireland, the Basque country and rural Brittany. Of western Ireland, Scheper-Hughes writes that: 'rural Ireland is dying' (1979) due to

The flight of young people – especially women – from the desolate parishes of the western coast, drinking patterns among the stay-at-home class of bachelor farmers, and the general disinterest [sic] of the local populace in sexuality, marriage and procreation are further signs of cultural stagnation.

(p. 4)

Scheper-Hughes (1979) argues that the shortage of marriageable women means that young farmers have no one to provide emotional attachment for them. Fox (1978: 91) reports a similar lack of young women on Tory Island off the Irish coast. Ballybran does come back to life in the summer holidays: 'Each summer in Ballybran the population of the parish is doubled by the seasonal return of village-born emigrants'. Older women told Scheper-Hughes that there had been little emotional satisfaction in their marriages:

Women of the younger generation are simply walking out on it. Over the past two decades, an average of twelve young women of marriageable age have left the village each year, contrasted to an average of four young men.

(1979: 108–109)

Girls leave with their mother's blessing: 'Did I want Aine to lead the life I had, stuck up here in the back of beyond with only the cows and the tea kettle for company?' (p. 109) one mother asked Scheper-Hughes rhetorically.

Scheper-Hughes's work on Ballybran caused a scandal, partly because of her statements that rural Ireland was dying, that the Gaelic revitalisation movement was failing, and partly because of her focus on the high levels of mental illness among bachelors in rural Ireland.

On a given research day in 1975 in the tiny parish of Ballybran . . . almost 5 per cent of the population of 461 people were receiving psychiatric care . . . Two-thirds of those patients were men, and all but one was single.

(1979: 65)

She argued that 'a residual population' (p. 71) is particularly vulnerable to mental illness, in particular schizophrenia. Her analysis of psychological and social stress in Ballybran has parallels with that of Favret-Saada's (1980) work in the countryside near

Paris, where failing farmers were prone to alcoholism and mental illness. The collapse of a rural social system with its casualties becoming mental patients is strikingly similar between the French Bocage and Ballybran.

Researchers in Germany have also reported a lack of enthusiasm for the role of farmer's wife among young women. In Golde's (1975: 117) two villages in south-west Germany he describes 'the Plight of the Bachelors'. In the Catholic village there was: 'a number of bachelor farmers with little hope of finding wives'. Twenty-eight per cent of farms were likely to cease operating due to a lack of wife and mother for the farmer. One bachelor told Golde:

> If I had a wife, everything could go on. So much has been invested in the farm and so far everything has worked out all right, but if my mother dies – I can't work the farm on my own.

Given the account Golde (1975: 114) provides of the woman's day which 'covers 15 hours or more. She is first to rise in the morning, and, after the evening meal when her husband grabs his coat and heads for the inn, she settles down to some more housework' women's lack of enthusiasm is hardly surprising.

McDonald (1989) found in rural Brittany that a common toast on New Year's Eve was: 'A happy New Year and may you find a lady wife before it is out.' Young Breton women were unenthusiastic about the isolated, dirty, physically demanding work that a farm needs. The only young women McDonald met who wanted to live on farms were highly educated, articulate, feminist, militantly Breton, 'back to the land', 'green' women, who did not fit the bachelor farmers' ideas about proper women.

The absence of brides for farmers is reported by Douglass (1975: 45) from the Basque country. He quotes a newspaper advertisement:

Looking for a Bride

A 36-year-old man, good farmer, self-employed, with his own house located near the plaza in a beautiful small town of Mixe. The young woman who would like to meet him may write to this newspaper in total confidence.

Douglass says that the bride famine is partly because life as a *baserritarrak* was felt to be inferior to town life, especially for women. In Echalar in 1968 the parish priest 'polled thirty eligible young ladies from *baserriak* as to their willingness to marry and remain on their natal farmsteads and received thirty negative replies' (1975: 53). This survey was done when the French economy was booming, so the young women could see a 'better' alternative, working in a French town for high (by Basque standards) wages. When the French economy is in recession a few women may choose rural life, as Rogers (1991) found in Ste Foy. When four girls from Echalar took a holiday on the Costa Brava together, they were signalling *to* Echalar that they were not going to be farmers' wives, as well as having a 'modern' holiday.

In the next section three exceptions to this flight from peripheral areas are examined: one in southern Italy, one in southern France and one in the Canary Islands.

Three exceptions to the rule: Locorontondo, Ste Foy and Los Santos

In the early 1970s Galt studied a tiny island – Pantellaria – off the coast of Sicily. In the early 1980s Galt settled in Locorontondo with his wife and son, to conduct a case study of an agrotown, Murgia dei Trulli, on the Apulian plateau where *trulli* (houses with domes rather like old fashioned conical beehives) are the traditional architecture. The book's title (Galt, 1991: 1) comes from a local proverb: 'If you want to eat bread, stay far from the church bells.'

Galt chose to study Locorontondo because the relative prosperity of the peasants and the settlement pattern are different from the stereotypical agrotown in the *mezzogiorno*. The 'typical' settlement was a hill town, with an impoverished peasant class trekking out to scattered plots of unproductive land each morning, frequently plots they rented or sharecropped from absentee landlords. Investment in agriculture was rare, in contrast to the *mezzadria* system of Umbria and other central and northern regions in Italy (see Silverman, 1968). In the stereotyped southern town, farmwork was loathed, and every opportunity to invest in property or business in the town was seized upon, further draining farming of capital. Several anthropologists have studied such hill towns and explained the poverty of the *mezzogiorno* in terms of absentee landlords, concentrated settlements, scattered plots, and lack of investment in the rented farm land. (See for example, Brogger, 1971; Davis, 1973; Schneider and Schneider, 1976.)

Galt (1991) chose Murgia dei Trulli because the peasants had moved out of the town to live on their land, and there is relative prosperity. By the time (the early 1980s) that Galt did his study, many of the men under 45 worked in a steel plant at Taranto, or as builders or in some other non-farming occupation, but they have their land, and still farm it with their wives' labour. Until the 1970s wine was the main product, which was shipped to the north of Italy to be made into Martini, Cinzano and other vermouths. Today most of the wine goes to a local co-operative winery to make a white wine sold mainly in Apulia.

Galt comments that in the Locorontondo there was no sign of the hatred for the soil and its associated toil that researchers elsewhere in southern Italy report. For example, Blok (1974: 48) was told that 'Manual work has been made by the devil.' In Locorontondo land is owned, and owned with pride, and work on a family's *own* land is done with satisfaction. Peasant families used to live in the town, but from 1810 onwards they began to move out into the country, and live *on* farms. Once out in the country they devised agricultural and social strategies for country life. All the forms of co-operation Banfield said did not exist in Montegrano did develop in Locorontondo – symbolised by the wine co-operative. Galt had discovered one of the pockets of prosperity and investment in southern Italy.

The second example is Ste Foy, in rural southern France. Susan Rogers (1985, 1991) had previously researched Grand Frault, a village in north-eastern France before studying Ste Foy. Between 1960 and 1975 Ste Foy had suffered a bride shortage. In these years young men were left owning farms but without wives. Ste Foy has the same single-heir system as Ballybran, and the son who inherited the *ostal* between 1960 and 1975 frequently found himself owning a farm but single, while other sons left the village and married. However, unlike Ballybran, Ste Foyans set about changing village life to make it attractive to potential brides.

> Most noticeably, beginning in the late 1960s, many began investing in home modernization and renovation. Previously, farm profits had generally been reinvested in the farm operation, while investments in the home or in raising standards of living were considered a great deal less important.
>
> (Rogers, 1991: 163)

As well as making material improvements, such as a modern kitchen, central heating, and so on, *ostals* changed work patterns so that a bride with a job continued it rather than being given uncongenial farm work (e.g. a nurse continued nursing and a pig man would be hired), or a business opportunity was created for the incoming wife to give her some autonomy. Rogers (1991: 164–165) tells the story of Sylvie and Colette who both left the village in the late 1970s, travelled to the UK, experienced non-farm work, but came back to marry Ste Foy men and inherit *ostals*, albeit of a 'reformed' kind. Unlike Ballybran, the social system in Ste Foy changed to encourage young women to return after a brief migratory experience, and the social system was stronger in 1989 than it had been in 1975.

The third example of a peripheral region changing to survive comes from the Spanish Canary Islands. Moore (1976b) is an account of the impact of foreign residents in a village on the Canary Islands. The village, Los Santos, Tenerife, in 1955 had 1,200 inhabitants struggling to live by farm work or fishing at the dry, barren end of the island. In a good year it rained three times; a dry spell with no rain at all could last four years. Three wealthy families owned all the farm land in a 20-kilometre radius and employed people from Los Santos to work in the tomato plots on the terraced slopes of the hills. Outsiders were rare, and few villagers ever travelled to the rest of the island. In 1956 a Swedish vet, dying of multiple sclerosis, found the village. He was looking for a cheap, warm, dry, isolated place to spend the rest of his life. Once settled in Los Santos, he suggested to six other crippled male Swedes he had met in hospital that they too came to the village.

During 1957 the seven men rented a house they called *Casa Sveca* (the Swedish House), organised Spanish lessons for themselves, and employed boys to push their wheelchairs, a cook and some maids. None of the men was rich in Swedish terms, but they were much better off than the landless villagers. Because they had money, the villagers were eager to sell them things they wanted. Enterprising people installed generators so that fridges and a film projector could be run. The local dressmakers started to make fashionable clothes for the women who came to visit the Swedes; the baker got a recipe for Swedish bread and started baking it; the fishermen began to run boat trips. Because the village had films, ice cream, rooms to let and a *pension* (developed originally to provide beds for the Swedes' visiting friends and relatives) tourists had something to come to, and began to bring more money to Los Santos. Young men in the village learnt about jobs in Holland and

Scandinavia, and were helped to go abroad to work by the Swedes. One man trained as a physiotherapist in Sweden and came back to work in the *Casa Sveca.*

This example of an isolated community transformed by the arrival of 'outsiders', yet not destroyed, because, Moore argues, the Swedes did not upset the local social structure, leads to the last theme of the chapter: tourism. In many EEC countries government sees tourism as the best solution to the problems of peripheral regions.

Is tourism the solution?

In all the countries with a peripheral region there is a body of opinion which argues that tourism is the best solution to the region's problems. There is, therefore, a conflict between the two future models of the future for the peripheral region. One is technocratic and rational, and is usually held by white-collar planners at the centre of the region or the country. The other is 'preservationist' or 'green', and is usually held by those who farm in the area, those in green parties and those who want to promote minority languages and cultures.

In the technocratic vision, peasants will be encouraged to abandon uneconomic land, and the countryside will be used for leisure instead. The peripheral area then provides recreation for the majority urban population, and jobs will be created for the displaced peasants. The technocratic model assumes the rural population will settle into tourist centres, where facilities can be provided. Opponents of these plans are either the peasants themselves – for whom land is not a commodity but a patrimony, a family trust – or those who wish to preserve the regional language and culture such as the Breton revivalists, or those who are hostile to the farming methods used in agri-business with lots of nitrates and weedkillers and want to return Europe to organic farming (e.g. Jenkins, 1979).

There are authors who do have faith in tourism as a 'solution', but they are outnumbered by doubters. Researchers such as Rosenberg, Reiter and Reiter (1973) have pointed out that:

1 Local peasants rarely have the skills, qualifications and certificates necessary to get the good jobs in tourist areas. For example to be a ski instructor you have to be not only a skilled skier but also have credentials.

2 Local peasants rarely have access to capital and credit, which are necessary to start businesses. To build a ski lift, or an hotel, or a theme park takes money.

The results of tourist development have not usually pleased anthropologists. Rosenberg, Reiter and Reiter say that in the south of France depopulation of rural areas has not been halted, farming has suffered, the social structure of the villages is upset, and there are new social tensions between 'old' locals and new élite outsiders. The case studies of Valloire by Susan and John Hutson (1971) support those of Rosenberg, Reiter and Reiter (1973). John Hutson (1971) presents a case study of a man – Martin – who wanted to build up tourism in Valloire. There was a conflict between the desire for wealth, new jobs and a halt to migration, and the standards and values of the moral community of the old Valloire. Valloire locals saw the village as a moral community where the insiders (the *gens du pays*) not only live in the village but share values. People outside Valloire are strangers (*étrangers*) who do not share the values. The belief system of the insiders is based on *égalité*, *indépendance* and *parenté* (equality, independence and kinship). The local slogan was that no-one was the boss of anyone else (*personne commande ici, nous sommes tous copains*). Independence means each family unit should be self-sufficient except for help from kin or neighbours with whom there are symmetrical helping relationships (*rendre service*). Families walked a narrow line between being independent and either indebted (*indetté*) which is bad, or too proud and stuck up. Martin tried to get a major ski investment to Valloire but he behaved like a stranger, broke the norms of the community, and was voted out of office. Valloire lost faith in him and hence the chance to be a ski resort.

The people in Abriès are equally polarised by tourism. Rosenberg (1988) reports that there had been some tourism in the Hautes-Alpes since 1900, but it was destroyed by the Second World War. In 1958 the Gaullist regime decided to promote winter tourism in the French Alps, and the people of Abriès were particularly hopeful that tourism would replace the jobs lost when Nestlés stopped buying milk in their area in 1970. Four hotels were opened, plus a caravan and camp site, a sanatorium which also provides ski holidays for Marseilles schoolchildren and a holiday home for retired working-class Parisians. In July, August and the height of the ski season Abriès is alive, the rest of the year it is not. The skiing appeals to working-class French people, and Rosenberg

(1988: 172–174) doubts whether anyone was making much profit from it. The man who makes real money from skiing came from Grenoble, and pays very low wages to the locals who work the lift and do other jobs. Rosenberg concludes: 'Cultivators assume that the hotel owners and local shopkeepers are making a profit from tourism. The shopkeepers and hotel owners assume that tourism benefits the cultivators' (p. 174). In fact, Rosenberg argues, neither is making much, and the two activities are not compatible. Like the peasants studied by Franklin (1969) Abriès is becoming a community of 'park-keeper peasants'.

Perhaps the oddest case of a tourist development upsetting the local social structure is Medjugorje. This village in the mountains of Hercegovina was poor, unknown and survived on the remittances of men working in Germany and Austria. On 24 June 1981 the Virgin Mary appeared to six children, and continued to do so every day thereafter for a decade. Fifteen million pilgrims and tourists visited Medjugorje in that decade, and changed the economy of the village completely. Bax (1991, 1992) is an account of how many women in the parish had developed what the local men (including the doctor and the priests) called *zenska histerija* (women's madness), which included perpetual exhaustion, agoraphobia, depression, vague fears of impending doom and paranoia. The women believed they were being sucked in by the *Crna Moca* (the Black Power), that is, that devils were possessing them. The men believed that the women were overworked because of the tourists, the women that the spiritual balance of the village had been disturbed. Bax is convinced that the social relations in the village had been radically changed, with negative consequences for both sexes.

This chapter has outlined the problems facing peripheral regions, and explored the possibilities of solving them by encouraging tourism.

SUGGESTED READING/ACTIVITY

Nancy Scheper-Hughes's (1979) *Saints, Scholars and Schizophrenics*, is an accessible book on a dying way of life: peasant farming.

Chapter 6

Towns with towers

The city as symbol and the neighbourhood as home

Beyond the seas are towns with towers. . .

(Flecker, 1947: 96)

INTRODUCTION

While the peripheral regions are full of smokeless homes, the cities grow and develop. This chapter deals with the research on every-day life in the cities of the EEC with more emphasis on the ordinary city-dwellers, rather than the élites or the middle classes. There are four main issues in this chapter:

1 the city or town as a symbol of a civilised lifestyle,
2 the pull of the urban area as a destination for migrants,
3 the research on everyday life in towns and cities,
4 the use of space in towns and cities by different classes and by men and women.

Before covering these four themes, it is important to recognise that anthropologists have been relatively neglectful of urban and town life compared to rural life, even though the majority of European people live in urban areas. Hansen (1987: 150) praised Michael Kenny (1960) because he had pioneered urban research in European anthropology.

> Prior to the publication of *A Spanish Tapestry*, few anthro-pologists had urbanites on their cognitive maps, and fewer still recognised that rural–urban relations were a fruitful vein of ethnographic inquiry.

Kertzer (1987: 152) made a similar point:

Michael Kenny was one of the pioneers in extending Mediterranean anthropology from mountain hamlets to cities, from the
agricultural to the urban. Recognising the centrality of the urban
experience . . . Kenny pointed anthropologists in new directions.

Kenny's original work on Madrid was not immediately copied.
Nearly twenty years after Kenny's study of Madrid, Davis (1977)
complained that the field was still dominated by rural studies, and
Crump (1975) objected strongly to the rural bias in the literature
by British and American researchers on Italy. Most of the contributors to the volume edited by Kenny and Kertzer (1983) made
the same points about the countries they knew.

Despite these calls for a more urban focus researchers still tend
to choose small villages as research sites (as I did for the hypothetical anthropologist Rachel Verinder in Chapter 1) and do not
explain or justify their choices. Parman (1990) chose a village in
the Outer Hebrides in 1970/71 and makes no apology for her
choice of such a marginal community in her book published
twenty years later. Makris (1992) chose a tiny Cretan village in
1978; O'Neill's (1987) Portuguese hamlet had only 187 inhabitants in 57 households when he went there in 1976; Stewart (1991)
chose a remote village on the Greek island of Naxos for his study
in 1983/84 and so on.

Not only have researchers continued to choose rural areas, it is
also striking that when anthropologists have studied a city, it is
frequently the same city. Thus we have several different accounts
of life in Seville (Press, 1979; Murphy, 1983a, 1983b; Marvin, 1988)
and in Barcelona (McDonogh, 1986a; Di Giacomo, 1987;
Pi-Sunyer, 1987; Woolard, 1989), but there are no English-
language studies published of Malaga, Toledo or Santander, or
other large Spanish cities. Similarly Athens has been studied by
several researchers (e.g. Hirschon, 1989; Kenna, 1990) but Thessa-
lonika and Patras have not been. Marseilles is an important migration destiny for rural French men and women in the southern half
of the country, but anthropologists have not produced ethnographies of it. In each European country it is easier to find an
account of life in a tiny village than in a provincial capital or major
industrial centre.

THE CITY AS 'CIVILISATION'

The town or city has a symbolic function as a centre of civilisation and of sin. Those who love cities praise their culture and excitement, those who loathe them despise the crowds, the anonymity and the wickedness. Every European country has its version of the folk tale about the town mouse and the country mouse. Those who belong to towns and cities regard themselves as superior *because* of their urbanity, even when their town is, to outsiders, tiny.

Silverman (1975) studied Montecastello di Vibio in central Italy, a town of 1,000 people. The inhabitants felt themselves to be sophisticated urbanities living in a city. Silverman reports that: 'The people of Montecastello are conscious of this quality of town life, indeed they glorify it . . . The Montecastellesi refer to themselves as *gente civile*' (p. 1). The Italian word *civilta* does not have an exact equivalent in English, because it carries the ideas of urbanity, civilisation, and 'civic-ness'. Similarly the inhabitants of Pisticci (Davis, 1973) chose to live in the agrotown because it was respectable and civilised to do so, even though it meant that the men had to trek miles to and from their fields every day. Town living is seen as better because the town is a place of learning, of smart clothes, of work that is clean and of living a respectable life under the watchful eye of neighbours. As Dundes and Falassi (1975) report for Siena, those 'born on the cobblestones' (*nati nelle lastre*) despise the peasants (*contadini*) who live outside Siena where the roads are not cobbled, metalled or paved.

The country-dweller may be seen as a bumpkin, an idiot who chews straw and is slow-witted and easily fooled, but he holds a parallel stereotype of the city slicker, whose very sophistication disadvantages him in the countryside. The tough, macho pastoralist such as the Sarakatsani (Campbell, 1964), Cretan shepherd (Herzfeld, 1985) or Sardinian mountain-dweller (Berger, 1986) despises the town-dweller as decadent and soft, fit only to be stolen from and outwitted. Similar stereotyping is reported between town and country in all European countries. For example Thornton (1987: 102) reports from Austria:

> mutual distrust and dislike is still tangible between country and city, and between labourer and professional. For example, the Viennese are maligned throughout the countryside as presumptuous aristocrats while the farmers are scorned by their metropolitan neighbours as country bumpkins.

Similarly in Malta, Boissevain (1965: 28) reported:

> The typical townsman was often described to me by villagers as
> a white-collar worker who goes to cocktail parties, tries to look
> like an Englishman – pipe, tweeds and moustache – and speaks
> English to his children. The villager, on the other hand, is
> portrayed as an illiterate rustic who spends his money on wine
> and fireworks, without a thought for the future of his children.

Both are caricatures, but both were held. In Italy Romanucci-Ross
(1991: 12) argues: 'To include a city in an area culture study is to
learn that urban design exhibits views of a moral ordering and
policies about personal and class interaction.' The moral ordering
is the sense of civilisation – a civilisation which is known to stretch
back a thousand, two thousand years. The researchers on Italy
have been particularly good at capturing the idea of the city as a
centre of civilised life, but the idea is equally prevalent in southern
Spain. As Corbin and Corbin (1987: 10) report: 'People in Ronda
are highly conscious of the fact that Ronda is in many ways
"superior" to the surrounding countryside.' People in Ronda know
that it is not a major city such as Malaga, Seville or Madrid, but it *is*
a town, not the countryside. Because it is a town, certain standards
are expected in dress and deportment. Tourists in the 1950s and
1960s violated these:

> local people objected to beachwear and other scanty summer
> clothing in town. Some tourists were arrested and fined for
> wearing shorts . . . sleeveless dresses or short skirts. Many
> foreigners assumed that the objection to exposed flesh
> reflected an antiquated sexual prudishness. In fact, what local
> people found most objectionable was not what was worn but
> where it was worn. The revealing clothing suggested that the
> tourists regarded the city as country and those who lived in it as
> uncultured.
>
> (Corbin and Corbin, 1987: 28)

THE PULL OF THE TOWN

As Hudson and Lewis (1985) point out, urban centres in all the
Mediterranean cultures are attracting young people, especially
young men, away from rural areas. This is partly because of the
idea that the urban area is a more civilised place to live, partly due

to economic pressures. Zonabend (1984: 90) reports that in Minot in Burgundy:

> Children not suitable for secondary education are the only ones left at the village school. All the others try for entry into secondary school at twelve or thirteen. If they are successful they become boarders and only return to the village at weekends or for the holidays. So the young people reach the town very early, and then get jobs that are essentially urban.

As Zonabend summarises it: 'there is a real thinning-out of this age-group over long periods' (p. 90).

Hudson and Lewis (1985: 17) argue that although there are difficulties in comparing patterns of internal migration:

> there does appear to have been a single dominant spatial pattern in Southern Europe over the past two generations. There has been an age and sex-selective rural to urban areas movement by young men in search of work and better living conditions.

This had led to 'a young concentration of the South European population in those major metropolitan areas, like Athens, Barcelona, Istanbul, Lisbon, Marseilles and Milan' (p. 18).

Hudson and Lewis argue that this migration has led to shanty towns, as illegal housing is built; and the conversion of rural 'under-employment into urban unemployment' (p. 18). A city like Athens (du Boulay, 1974), Barcelona (Pi-Sunyer, 1987) or Marseille (Rosenberg, 1988) is an attractive alternative to village life. The urban areas suffer housing shortages, 'solved' by illegal, substandard building, and unemployment. The rural areas become increasingly feminised, poorer, less powerful, and hence receive even fewer services.

RESEARCH METHODS IN CITIES AND TOWNS

The methods used by generations of anthropologists to study villages and rural areas outlined in Chapter 1, are clearly problematic in towns and impossible in cities. When Rosenberg (1988) lived in Abriès there were fewer than 200 people in 'the highest inhabited valley in Europe' (p. 1), when Just (1991) went to Spartohori in 1977 it had a population of 187 households, many with only one person in them, so he could meet every single person and everyone knew everyone else. When Kenna (1990) went to Nisos in 1966 the island's population was about 400, so she could be a familiar sight for all the islanders and include all of them in her research.

These are not feasible strategies in urban areas or even in small towns. The Corbins (1987) for example, point out that Ronda had about 17,000 inhabitants when they went there in 1966, and by 1979 had 30,000. When they began their fieldwork – which they have spent twenty years doing on and off – Ronda was already too big for them to meet everyone, and like many European towns and cities, it is growing rapidly. Quite a small town can have far too many inhabitants for a pair of anthropologists to meet or even observe.

To understand how researchers go about studying in an urban area, it is necessary to draw a contrasting example of a piece of research to go with the Galician village study invented for Chapter 1. Imagine that Rachel Verinder starts her PhD alongside a fellow student Franklin Blake, who is passionately committed to urban anthropology and determined to study city life. When Rachel sets off for her Galician fishing village, Franklin packs his bags and heads for Munich. Here he is likely to settle on one of three strategies to find a manageable project. He could choose a neigh-bourhood and live in it, and treat it as an urban village as Press (1979) did in Seville. He could choose one set of people, such as migrants from a particular place and make them his focus as Grillo (1985) did in Lyon, and Kenny (1960) did in Madrid. He could choose an institution or organisation, such as a hospital or a factory, and treat that as a microcosm of the city. This is frequently done by urban anthropologists in America, such as the contrib-utors to the collections edited by Messerschmidt (1982) and Burawoy and his colleagues (1991). Alternatively, Franklin could choose one category of people, such as members of a trade union, or tour guides, or priests, or practitioners of acupuncture, or antique dealers, and focus on them (see for example Sheehan, 1993, on the Dublin intellectuals). McKevitt's (1991a, 1991b) work in San Giovanni Rotondo focused on devotees of Padre Pio, a sub-group of the population of that town; and McDonogh (1986a) focused on the 'Good Families' in Barcelona, between a hundred and two hundred elite families in a city of 2 million inhabitants.

Munich has neighbourhoods, both blocks of flats and streets of houses near the centre, plus suburbs. It has migrants from Greece, Italy, Vietnam, Turkey, Yugoslavia and the former East Germany, as well as Germans who have moved in from the rural areas or other centres in Germany. Franklin could therefore choose all sorts of projects for his PhD in Munich, and settle down to use the same range of methods, or a selection of them, as Rachel uses in her fishing village. He could even focus on Bavarian separatists to parallel her Galician regionalists. Munich will be much more expensive, and might be full of distractions for a scholar, but anthropology is still possible and rewarding. The fieldwork contexts will be more varied in a big city, depending on the project. McDonogh (1986a: xi) describes doing fieldwork at the opera:

> families invited me into another experience of the opera house in the aristocratic loges of the first balcony. The first performance I saw from this vantage was Montserrat Caballe singing *L'Africane* in her home theatre. The magnificence of that performance highlighted the dualities of my role as participant observer – half attentive to the stage and half attentive to the dramas around me.

Compare that fieldwork setting with Belmonte's Naples. Belmonte (1983: 275) lived in a district he calls Fontana del Re:

> The district was notorious in Naples as a dangerous zone, a den of thieves, roughnecks, and prostitutes . . . a disproportionate number of the inhabitants earned their living collecting cardboard and junk.

Not at all like the opera house in Barcelona.

Kenny and Kertzer (1983) contains chapters which give overviews of the research done on urban life in Spain by Kenny and Knipmeyer (1983), on Italy by Kertzer (1983), on Greece by Vermuelen (1983) and on Yugoslavia by Spangler (1983). There is a need for similar synopses of English-language material on urban life in Portugal, France, Ireland, Denmark, Germany, Belgium, Holland and even the UK, for which the two syntheses (Frankenberg, 1966, and Bell and Newby, 1971) are both badly dated.

Fieldwork in urban settings can present problems for the researcher, and for the readers of the research. The dangers of adopting the world view of the particular sub-group chosen for study and then presenting it as the world view of the whole city are real ones. Thus Gilmore (1985) has criticised the Corbins (1983, 1987) for concentrating on the middle class in Ronda and not making it clear enough that life there is very different for a gypsy or a poor person. The view of life in Naples gained by Belmonte via his flat in a slum and his informants who were the family of a rubbish collector (Belmonte, 1979, 1989) is a partial one, not always put in perspective by the author. The lack of balance can be a problem for the reader when there is only one study of a city, or where the other work is similarly focused. Pardo (1989) has also worked in inner-city Naples, in 1978–80, but also on the poorest inhabitants and the most widely available paper is on death and mortuary practices, so does not provide a counter-balance to Belmonte's view on family life, crime, poverty and the labour market. We need an ethnography of middle-class residents in Naples too.

EVERYDAY LIFE IN TOWNS AND CITIES

In this section the material on four populations which have been studied by anthropologists which give insights on four different aspects of life in urban areas is explored. The research on an indigenous, long-established 'ethnic' minority in a city by Moore (1976a), on a working-class neighbourhood by Press (1979), on the elite of Barcelona by McDonogh (1986a) and on recent immigrants to a French city by Grillo (1985) is summarised to illustrate various facets of life in towns.

Bearing in mind the problems facing a researcher who wants to study urban life, and the dangers of mistaking the outlook of the chosen sub-group for that of all the city-dwellers, the research that has been done can be explored. One theme urban researchers have been concerned with is how far city life is different from rural life in the same society. Are issues of social control, of the protection of women, of kinship, of practical religion, of housework, of childrearing the 'same' in a city as they are in the countryside?

The first example is a case study of an indigenous minority, who had lived in the same city for 500 years, invisible to any outsider. In exploring their lives, Moore also explores life in Palma, Mallorca. It is also an example of a carefully presented piece of research, because the author studied a tiny sub-culture, but is meticulous in his presentation of them *as* a minority, and does not try to suggest they are representative of the whole city. Moore (1976a) studied one of the most odd-sounding urban groups – the Catholic Jews of Mallorca – the Xuetas. He was living in Mallorca when he stumbled onto the existence of this outcast group, stereotyped by other

Mallorquins as having bad manners, being dirty, ugly and clannish. To an outsider like Moore, a non-Mallorquin, the Xueta were completely invisible, and once he focused on them, the negative stereotype of the Xueta dissolves for the reader. They are actually an eminently respectable, middle class, devoutly Catholic, set of shop owners, exactly the sort of group anthropologists often neglect. The Xueta used to live in one street of silver shops (Calle de Plateria) in Palma, kept jewellery shops and lived in the flats above them. This was their neighbourhood. They were comfortably off, even rich. The Xuetas are good Catholics, have been for centuries, keep old-fashioned Mallorquin customs and are endogamous (that is, they marry inside their community not with outsiders). Their distant ancestors converted to Catholicism from Judaism in the fifteenth century.

In 1965 Moore set out to study the Xuetas. He found an informant Miguel Forteza, who had pride in being a Xueta and pride in assimilation of the Xueta into the mainstream of Mallorquin life. Such a person is called a 'key informant' or a 'gatekeeper', and is particularly useful in urban ethnography when the researcher needs help to meet the members of a particular sub-culture.

By the 1960s not all the Xueta were still running businesses as gold and silversmiths, and not all still lived in 'their' street. Some had other businesses, some lived elsewhere in Palma. However, when Moore studied them in 1965 Xueta men still regularly met in 'their' street in one of the bars/coffee shops where their circle of friends (*tertulia*) was centred, whether they lived and worked there or not. The Xueta had their own church – St Eulalia's – in their *barrio*, with a Xueta priest, and their own cofraternity (the Cross of Calvary) to march in the Holy Week procession. Even Xueta who lived away from their neighbourhood returned on Sundays and feast days to worship at St Eulalia's. Historically, they had not been welcome at other churches, and had to have their 'own' church with their 'own' priest. Moore (1976a) is quite convinced that there is no doubt of the Xueta's devout Catholicism, but despite their public Catholicism, other non-Xueta Mallorquins whispered to Moore, 'Are they Roman Catholics or really (secretly) still Jews?' From the perspective of the non-Xueta Mallorquin, the Xuetas are a pariah sub-cultural segment.

Moore found that the Xueta identity was still strong. They called themselves *'d'es carrer'* or *'los de la calle'*, which both mean 'Those of the street', rather than using the word Xueta, and were proud of their separate sub-culture. To a Spanish-speaker from outside Mallorca, of course, the sentence 'I'm of the street' would be meaningless, while to a Xueta it was a statement of belonging.

In 1965 the 4,718 Xueta were 3–4 per cent of the population of Palma, and were middle-class entrepreneurs. Moore wanted to test the statement that they were endogamous, and devised an ingenious research strategy using the telephone directory. He became aware that Xueta had distinctive surnames, different from those common to other Mallorquins. He discovered a set of fifteen surnames, common in the 'Silver' street, and therefore identifiably Xueta. Because of the Spanish naming system, people carry surnames of both their parents. So when Maria Garcia de Perez marries Arturo Rodriguez de Guzman she becomes Maria Garcia de Rodriguez. So if people have two of the fifteen Xueta names they are examples of Xueta endogamy. Moore found from the telephone book that there was 70 per cent endogamy. The Xueta had strong *barrio* loyalty and did indeed marry each other rather than other Mallorquins, partly because other Mallorquins would not marry a Xueta.

By the time Moore came to write about the Xueta he felt that the changes currently affecting Mallorca would continue to affect them. As tourism boomed, many non-Mallorquin Spaniards came to live in the island and they had no knowledge of, or prejudice against, Xueta. To outsiders all Mallorquins were 'the same', the Xueta were indistinguishable from the rest. As the Xueta move out of their old visible *barrio* the distinctions between Xueta and other Mallorquins are no longer marked. Spanish immigrants marry Xuetas and non-Xueta Mallorquins and all become a *mélange*, so that endogamy is declining. Most Xueta were bourgeois Mallorquins, and shared with other Mallorquins an ambivalence about the merits of traditional Mallorquin life versus the status of modern European life which was increasingly available to bourgeois people in Palma. The urban citizens of Palma, Xueta and non-Xueta, had, until the 1960s, shared a disdain for rural life which was scorned as 'peasant' life. In the mid-1960s, having a bit of land and a house in country for weekends was an important middle-class status symbol – and a symbol of a person's identity and attachment to traditional Mallorquin way of life which marked them off from other non-Mallorquin Spaniards and foreigners. Xueta and non-Xueta were adopting this middle-class status symbol, the country house.

The case study of the Xueta is unusual because they are middle class, an outcast minority, and a group whose life was being changed by tourism in a city. When Moore wrote his book there was a plan to demolish the old city of Palma, including the Xueta *barrio*, and he was sure that they would vanish when their street was knocked down. In fact the old quarter of Palma has not been demolished, and in 1989 there was still a street of jewellers with St Eulalia's Church at one end. Xueta names could be found on shops there, but also on other businesses all over Palma. The most interesting feature of the Xueta case study is the way in which the arrival of non-Mallorquin Spaniards meant Xueta/non-Xueta distinctions were less important than they had been for 500 years.

One of the badges of devotion to Catholicism displayed by the Xueta was modelling the cofraternity (the Cross of Calvary) on its original in Seville, and going there to ensure their costumes for the Holy Week Parade were authentic. Holy Week in Seville is:

> among Christendom's greatest shows. All Seville turns out for days of passionate display, as fifty-three *cofradias* wind their ways through impossibly narrow streets . . . most *cofradias* contain members of all social strata . . . Holy Week is a convincing display of wealth, well being, solidarity, and continuity.
>
> (Press, 1979: 24–25)

It is to Press's account of life in a working-class *barrio* of Seville that the chapter now turns. One type of dwelling in Seville is the *corral de vecinos* (literally a corral of neighbours). This is a building with one street entrance and a patio, onto which front lots of one-room flats, let at low rents, and with shared lavatories. In 1970 there were 2,000 such corrals, each housing about twenty families, usually of four people. So Press suggests that 160,000 Sevillanos out of 600,000 lived in corrals in 1970 when he began his research. Many of them have nicknames (Corral of the Sausage) and Press studied one he calls the Corral of the Wet Widow (after a widow who drowned herself in the Guadalquivir river). There are twenty-two flats, half with one room, half with two. People cook in the patio or outside their doors, there are communal basins, a shower, two lavatories and a tap of drinking water in the patio. Press gives pen portraits of the inhabitants of the corral, who are a mixture of people who have always lived there, some who have fallen on hard times and others on their way up and out. Half the residents had lived there for more than twenty years, nine had been there thirty-five years or more. Press summarises the majority of inhabitants as: 'a city-wise, gregarious, locally-raised population of steady though low-wage earners' (1979: 66).

All the rooms can be seen by the residents of all the others, so the thirty-five adults and fifteen children have little privacy. Gossip is rife and quarrels always a possibility. Press was able to collect detailed family budgets, and shows how different families and households in the Wet Widow balance or fail to balance their finances. Some are saving to get out of the corral, others spend what they earn. Press shows how lotteries are a vital part of life and so is credit.

> Young Margrita pays 20 pesetas weekly to a shoe store whether she buys or not. At any time she can purchase shoes there to a total of 600 pesetas and continue paying only 20 per week. Each week the shop holds a drawing. Winners receive a paid-up chit for 600 pesetas.
>
> (1979: 232)

The financial abilities of some of the residents are considerable. Alberto had a brother who was a taxi-driver in Seville, but went to Germany as a guestworker, leaving Alberto to drive the taxi. After eight years the brother returned, and sat down with Alberto and his other two brothers to decide on an investment. They settled on a bar. They heard about a new block of flats being put up, bought one for their aged mother, and built their bar in the development. So the four of them could run a business and see their mother. The bar has flourished, as no others exist among these new flats, and Alberto expects to be able to get his family out of the Wet Widow.

Press also deals at some length with religious behaviour, kinship, health and illness, and sex and gender. He found that the behaviour of women was policed *more* strictly than in villages. Women can only avoid gossip by staying close to home:

> and on those daily occasions when they must go shopping, they prefer to go in pairs, or, at the very least, with a child in tow. Any child will do, and corral women regularly take neighbours' daughters along to the market. Men do not force women to behave in this manner. Women are as committed to maintaining a reputation of honour as are their men.
>
> (1979: 136)

The life Press describes is urban, but essentially small-scale. People move in a circle of kin and friends, using contacts to get jobs, get flats, get through the bureaucracy, and gossiping about their relatives and neighbours. The working-class *barrio* is as much a 'village' as any of the real villages studied by rural anthropologists. Thuren (1988) is a parallel study in Valencia. Press also gathered information on middle- and even upper-class Sevillanos, and contrasts life in the Wet Widow with that in smart modern flats and ancestral town houses. The reader is given a rounded picture of life in Seville, omitting only the gypsies (outcasts) and the poorest inhabitants: those who have migrated to Seville and not yet established themselves with networks of kin, friends and neighbours who can get them jobs, flats and help them hassle the bureaucracy.

Press's vivid account of life in the Wet Widow can be contrasted with McDonogh's work in a bigger, industrial Spanish – or rather Catalan – city: Barcelona. McDonogh (1986a, 1987) has studied both the élite families of Barcelona and written about its most notorious neighbourhood, the *barrio chino*. His book-length work on the élite families is a rare contribution to European anthropology because it is not about the poor, the immigrants or an oddity like the Xueta.

The 'Good Families' of Barcelona are about a hundred to two hundred families, with between 2,000-3,000 members who have controlled the economy of Catalonia for 150 years. McDonogh shows how wealth, intermarriage between élite families, education and a clear sense of class membership serve to keep the élite apart from the rest of the population of Barcelona. They have followed the Catalan custom of a single heir, so that wealth is not dissipated or divided. The single heir, either a son (*hereu*) or daughter (*pubilla*), gets at least three-quarters of the total estate, and the remaining quarter is divided equally between *all* the heirs including the *hereu*. Daughters are expected to use their share as a dowry, non-inheriting sons to establish themselves in a career. The heir's marriage contract settles all the legacies, and McDonogh was able to consult such contracts in the city archives, tracing how families preserved their farms in the eighteenth century, and factories in the nineteenth and twentieth. He presents the history of the Guells from 1800–1980. The modern élite family starts with Juan Guell Ferrer who returned from Cuba in 1836 and invested his wealth in a textile factory, and later a bank and a machine-tool firm. Juan served in Parliament, and was active in lobbying for Catalan industry. His son Eusebio was the main heir, expanded the business and was a patron of the architect Gaudi. Eusebio diversified into railways, insurance and, through his wife, tobacco. He was made a Count, consolidating the family's position in the Barcelona élite. His chief heir was Juan Antonio, the eldest son of ten children, who died in 1955. The head of the family in Barcelona at the time of McDonogh's research had built on the success of the second Eusebio, who had married the heiress to a Catalan shipping fortune. In 1980 the Guells were major industrialists and cultural patrons, and active in Catalan politics.

The lives of such families are spent intertwined. They go to the same schools, worship at the same churches, attend the same classes at the same university, marry each other, discuss each other and share the same social life. As two symbols of their separateness McDonogh focuses on the Liceu (the Opera House) and the Old Cemetery. The Opera House was built in the 1840s, and has seats on six floors, the ground level and five balconies. The first balcony (*planta noble*) is the most exclusive, with a wide passageway where people can parade between the acts. The *planta noble* and the next two floors are for the richest people, while the upper balconies are for: 'those of limited resources, who might otherwise not hear any opera: students, artisans or workers' (McDonogh, 1986a: 193).

The Good Families own boxes on the ground floors, in one case a box they have owned since 1844, and the ownership of a box is always mentioned in the will of the family head and left to the main heir. If a family gives up its opera box, it is publicly withdrawing from the Catalonian élite. When a death occurred a family closed its box at the opera for the rest of the season, and, as late as the 1950s, appearing in evening dress at the opera was the sign that a young woman had left the schoolroom and was available for marriage.

If the Good Families display themselves while alive at the opera, after death their élite status is maintained in the Old Cemetery. When built in 1819 this had three sections: a paupers' ditch, a middle area with wall niches and an inner area with mausolea for the élite families. These mausolea could hold ten to twelve coffins at the same time. When full, the tomb is closed and a new one built. As late as the 1920s it was fashionable to parade round these tombs on 2 November, the Feast of All Souls, as a social event which was written up in the society pages.

It may seem odd to look to the graveyard for symbolism about the living, but Barcelona is not alone. In Locorontondo class distinctions in the town are marked in life and in death. Galt (1991) describes the town cemetery. The élite families have elaborate tombs in the centre of the cemetery, the poor are buried in communal tombs that line the walls. As Galt puts it 'Élite landowners and professionals occupied the centre of the cemetery just as they occupied the centre of town life' (p. 63).

These two places: the opera and the Old Cemetery provided an opportunity for the élite to see and be seen, to reaffirm their social status in Barcelona. More studies of such élites in other European cities are needed before the Good Families of Barcelona can be contrasted with non-Catalan, non-industrial élites.

The final example of an urban ethnography is a return to poor people, in this case the North African immigrants in Lyon. Grillo (1985) lived in Lyon in 1974–76 with his family, and studied the lives of North African immigrants and the response of Lyon to them. It is clear that the arrival of the North Africans revealed many things about Lyon, and it was easier to study the 'structural response of French society to immigrants' (p. 20) than the lives of the immigrants themselves. It was also more revealing. That is, more facets of urban life are made apparent when an 'alien' group arrives and makes things problematic.

The lives of North African immigrants in Lyon are much harder than those of the working-class inhabitants of the Seville *barrio* studied by Press (1979). They have the worst jobs in the labour market, the worst housing, and if they have their families with them their lives are scrutinised by social workers, and their children fail in the schools. The labour market is segregated so that 'French' French people get the nicest jobs (and all those in government service which are restricted to French nationals), then the Italians and Spaniards, with the North Africans doing the dirtiest, least skilled and most insecure jobs. Many of the North Africans are men on their own, living in hostels. These are cheap, and mean men are among other Muslims in a similar predicament, but behaviour is policed: political activity is forbidden for example. Grillo found that some men had been hostel-dwellers for many years: 'In one hostel I met two Algerians who had stayed there since 1954' (1985: 103). That is twenty years in the same hostel, broken only by summer trips 'home' each year. Men in hostels are usually trying to save as much as possible to send home, and to invest when they return. A hostel director told Grillo:

> They do not go out much in the evening or at weekends. They
> sit in the hall, or in their own rooms, drinking coffee and

playing cards. There are some residents I have never even seen watching television.

(1985: 105)

If a North African man does decide to bring his family over he faces bureaucratic hurdles, and then housing is a major problem. Ironically, many North African families start off in blocks of flats built in the 1960s to house *pieds noirs* when they came home from Algeria. The *pieds noirs* quickly left these grim flats, and were replaced by Tunisian, Moroccan and Algerian families. Grillo summarises the state of these flats: 'To say that Simon skimped on their construction would be more than generous' (p. 116). (Simon was the builder.) Better housing is expensive, hard to find, and few landlords want to let to North Africans. One problem is that flats were built for families with two children and many North African families have five, or even ten.

Much of Grillo's book consists of middle-class French – teachers, social workers, union officials, politicians – describing their attempts to 'help' the North Africans become *évolué* (evolved, civilised): that is *French*. Baffled family planning experts try to cut family size; home economists try to change diet; housing workers try to change cleaning methods; educationalists run Arabic classes for the French and French classes for the North Africans. These are all well-meaning people, not the racists who want everyone sent home, but they are totally convinced that the sooner the Algerian woman abandons Islam, speaks French, takes the Pill, gets a job, and stops cooking *couscous* her life will be better: the closer she becomes to a French urban woman the happier she will be. There is no recognition that anyone might want to work in Lyon but *stay* Algerian.

In Lyon the social workers and teachers were equally worried about the Portuguese, who were also regarded as '*sauvages*' (savages) because they had come from rural areas without plumbing, electricity and were illiterate. (Italian and Spanish guestworkers were not seen as problems in the same way.) The overall picture Grillo produces is one of an underclass, partly created by prejudice, partly by misunderstandings. The second-generation North Africans face worse problems than their parents, for they have higher expectations but leave the French school system no better qualified than their fathers, to meet a hostile labour market. (The collection of papers edited by Wilpert (1988a) deals with this problem throughout Europe.)

With these four urban studies we have the beginnings of an anthropology of city life in Europe. This chapter now briefly deals with two further, related, topics: class and gender issues in the city and the research on the uses of space in urban areas.

CITY SPACE: CLASS AND GENDER DIFFERENCES MADE VISIBLE

The final theme of this chapter is the research on how different groups use city spaces. Often a researcher can find out about class and gender differences in cities by watching which groups utilise which parts of the area, at which times of the day, at which seasons of the year, how they move in them and how they dress.

If Franklin Blake, our imaginary researcher in Munich, wanted to get a sense of the class and gender pattern of the neighbourhood in which he has found a flat, one way to do it is to watch the people coming and going. If he lived near Rosenheimer Platz he could start his day in a cafe near the entrance to the underground station which opens at 6 a.m. (Monday to Friday) to sell breakfast (with beer if you want it) to local men on their way to work. At 6 a.m. people are leaving on the underground trains, not arriving, and the men are in clothes suitable for manual work. Later men in business suits appear, schoolchildren pass, the trains start disgorging men and women in suits who work near here, women come out shopping. Greek, Turkish, Italian and German can be heard: there are women in twos and threes with their heads covered and women alone in jeans. Just by sitting and watching and listening Franklin could get a sense of Munich as a city with several social classes, several different guestworker groups, different standards of female behaviour and so on.

Herzfeld (1991: 3) does an analysis of this type on smell in old Rethemnos.

> Early in the morning, above the fading dankness of the night, the warm spiceness of baking bread announces a long-established local craft. Another craft answers as, with the shrilling of their equipment, the carpenters' sawdust adds a distinctive sharpness, later drowned in the still more nostril-dilating acridity of varnish. As the shadows shorten towards late morning, the . . . sweetness of warming olive oil, wafted from dark windows, draws rich savour from meat, tomato, garlic and

onion . . . The narrow streets have begun to reverberate to the screech and roar of motorbikes and the impatient horns of trucks . . . Finally, with the leisurely, strolling tourists come[s] the chemical scent of suntan oil, from, especially, the foreign women now heading for the beach . . .

In this extract Herzfeld brings alive the populations using old Rethemnos, locals and tourists. Urban researchers can often 'see' the class differences that exist in urban areas and in small towns, which are more visible in towns and cities. Galt's (1991) work on Locorontondo, in Apulia, reveals the class inequalities of the town. He shows a major difference between the class system of the town and that of the countryside. The town had a full range of social classes, from élite landowners to beggars. The countryside was only populated by peasants all the year round, living in patriarchal extended families, and is now occupied by what Galt calls the 'postpeasants' living in nuclear families. Galt's interest was in explaining why the postpeasant family was able to develop in the countryside, away from the class domination of the urban élite, and thus escaped the *misería* of other cultivators in the *mezzogiorno*. His answer is that a combination of land tenure, a market for the grapes, and 'their extraordinary motivation to work until their bones ached' (p. 242), helped the postpeasants to develop a richer life than counterparts elsewhere in southern Italy. In the rural areas the class system of southern Italy is not visible, in the town it is readily apparent, in the clothes, the housing and the burial places of the rich. By leaving the town to live in the country the peasants partially escaped the domination of the upper class not only symbolically but in practice.

Class differences in the use of space are readily apparent in Spanish towns and cities. Gilmore's (1980) study of an Andalusian agrotown shows how the upper classes live in a different style of house, spend their time in different parts of the town and, symbolically, at festival times they meet other elite inhabitants in private pavilions, not out on the streets in public view. The Corbins' (1987) analysis of housing and space in Ronda is a parallel study of how middle class, working class and gypsies live in quite separate neighbourhoods in different types of housing.

Another approach to studying urban life is to discover the 'mental maps' people have of their town or city: that is, how they picture their environment. In large towns and cities many people may never see large tracts of the urban area. Classes may well live in one neighbourhood and work in another and have no reason to go anywhere else. Many of the studies in urban areas have focused on neighbourhoods, because they may be the limit of the social world for their inhabitants and function as face-to-face communities exactly 'like' villages. In Britain, Young and Wilmott (1957) reported this for a London neighbourhood, Bethnal Green. Dundes and Falassi (1975) show that in Siena the seventeen *contrada* have such loyal members so hostile to other *contrade*, that the territories are like little city states within Siena.

In many cities particular neighbourhoods may be 'home' to immigrants from a particular area. In Athens arrivals from a particular island such as Nisos (Kenna, 1990) congregate in one neighbourhood, the refugees from Turkey are still in their area (Hirschon, 1989) and so on. Sontz (1987) has studied Nordstadt, an industrial neighbourhood on the outskirts of a Germany city, which has a glass factory that has attracted migrant workers. In the nineteenth century workers came to Nordstadt from rural areas of Germany, in the 1950s and 1960s migrants came from southern Italy. In 1974 there were 806 Italians in Nordstadt, one-third of the population of the neighbourhood. However, because the German and Italian workers were employed in different parts of the glassworks, and on different shifts, they rarely met and certainly did not mix socially. The two groups were not on the streets at the same times of the day or on the same days of the week. Similar findings are reported by Yucel (1987) who studied the Turkish guestworkers in Offenbach. He and his wife went to Germany without work permits, and took jobs 'illegally' – without work permits. Yucel worked in a jeans workshop, run by a Turk, staffed by a mix of Turks, Yugoslavs, Greeks and Italians. Each group lived among others of the same race, religion, language and nationality, and used their networks among others of the same ethnic group to find jobs, flats and mutual help. When the German government started tightening up on 'illegal' workers in 1972 the networks were used to warn employees that the police were coming on raids searching for 'illegals'. These Turks had 'their' Offenbach which was quite different from that of non-Turks in Offenbach.

There are also different patterns of space usage by males and females. In traditional southern European cultures, public spaces are for men. Men sit and stand in the streets and the squares, men walk across squares when they need to. Women are expected to stay at home, leaving only for shopping and church. If a woman has to cross a square she will walk round the edge, close to the buildings, not saunter across the open space. Respectable women do not stand on street corners or sit in the town or neighbourhood square, they stand or sit on their own doorsteps. This relation between gender and space is discussed in more detail in Chapter 9.

CONCLUSIONS

Town and city life is the norm for most of the population of the EEC. It has not been studied enough, so many aspects of city and town life are not documented. The research we do have makes it clear that urban life is very different for various social classes, for males and females, for the rich and the poor, and that urban life is not necessarily anonymous and private: it can be just as tightly policed by gossip and kinship as any village.

SUGGESTED READING/ACTIVITY

Press (1979), *The City as Context*, gives a vibrant account of Seville.

Chapter 7

And with great lies

Politics, patronage and leadership

> That talkative, bald-headed seaman came
> . . . From Troy's doom-crimson shore,
> And with great lies about his wooden horse
> Set the crew laughing. . .
>
> (Flecker, 1947: 138)

INTRODUCTION

Ulysses/Odysseus may seem a remote ancestor of Jean Monet or Jacques Delors, yet the heroic leader of the Greeks against the Trojans has some characteristics in common with politicians in contemporary Europe. Cynicism about leaders is captured in the chapter title, as it is in the proverb from Agnone (Douglass, 1984: 192): 'He who engages in politics, engages in dirt' (*Chi fa politica, fa schifo*).

There are six themes in this chapter. First, factions, then local patronage and leadership, and then the impact of national politics on local communities. The chapter then turns to the inequalities in societies which make some people patrons and leaders and others clients and followers. There is a discussion of stratification, of élites, and of the values which leaders and patrons must have to be admired in their own communities. Throughout the chapter it will be apparent that in some communities politics is a matter for men, whether at the level of local patronage *or* national politics; while in others local patronage is very much a matter for women, even when national politics are a man's world. Finally, the links between politics and religion are briefly mentioned, and the topic of mafia and bandits fitted into the picture.

FACTIONS

In many small communities politics is a matter of factions. The hamlet, village or neighbourhood is divided into opposing parties or factions. These may be stable over many generations or constantly shifting. Their basis may be economic, or religious, or familial, or linguistic, or some incident now wrapped in myth. In Torbel, Netting (1981) found there were two factions, which had existed for at least fifty years. In local 'history' they had their origins when a man went to church in an overcoat (an item of city, middle-class clothing) and an opponent blew his nose on it. Descendants of the two sides were still opposed on every issue, and the feud was inherited. Netting was told, (1981: 190) 'One is born into a party'.

The factional allegiances determined which of the two groceries one shopped in, which political party was supported in national elections, and whether one became involved in the *Alte Musik* village band (fifes and drums) or the *Neue Musik* (brass instruments). Netting watched the village square for a period and says that it was possible to map the men's allegiances according to which other men they greeted and which they 'cut'.

A similar division existed in the Maltese village, Hal Farrug, studied by Boissevain (1965, 1969, 1984) where there were two factions supporting opposed saints: Saint Martin and Saint Rocco (Saint Roque). Each faction centred on a band club, which organised the celebration (*festa*) for their saint's day. The two *partiti* had been hostile to each other for eighty years when Boissevain first went to Malta in 1960. In 1877 everyone in Hal Farrug had supported St Martin, but then a new priest Don Rokku came, from a village where St Roque was the patron saint, and he started a confraternity for 'his' favourite saint. The village divided into two groups, one loyal to St Martin, the other choosing to support St Roque. Ever since 1877 the village had been divided. Those who were adherents of one faction joined one band club and shunned the other. 'Neutrals' paid dues to both band clubs and tried not to get involved. Boissevain found that most people followed their parents into one or the other faction, and married within it. One man who had been a St Roque supporter got engaged to the daughter of the President of the St Martin club, and was forced to change factions in order to marry the girl. The division was so strong in Hal Farrug that it polarised school children's clothing.

For example, a former head teacher of the Farrug School told me that he once tried to get the girls to wear the dark blue hair ribbons which are supposed to be part of their school uniforms. He was astounded when half the girls flatly refused. It was then explained to him that blue is the colour of the St. Roque *partito*, so the St. Martin girls could not be expected to wear it.

(Boissevain, 1965: 87)

The factions competed to have bigger processions, let off bigger fireworks and be 'better' in village life. The St Martin club had celebrated its centenary in 1960 with a big *festa*, so in 1978 the St Rocco supporters celebrated theirs with a massive show of loyalty. (Boissevain, 1984: 129). In 1979 schoolgirls whose families were of the St Martin faction would still wear hair-ribbons of the correct colour (red) and those supporting St Rocco would wear blue.

In Grand Frault (Lorraine) Rogers (1991: 118) found that there were two factions, and it was easy to discover whether a new acquaintance was in one or the other. One faction called her 'Suzanne', the other 'Suzie', so the name used by a new contact immediately told Rogers which network they belonged to.

In Ambeli before the coup of 1967 there were two factions, one Left and one Right, who met in different cafés. The two owners were enemies, and choosing which café to use meant declaring support for one man or the other (du Boulay, 1974: 225). In local politics issues and divisions can last for many years – even generations. In the Catholic village studied by Golde (1975: 146) there were still, in 1970, 'Nazi' and 'anti-Nazi' factions which went back to the 1930s. A fight at one of the inns in 1970 was seen as trouble between the factions. In Abriès, there was a factional dispute which went back at least twenty years. One faction supported Jean Alland, a former mayor. They shop at his grocery, sit near him in church and greet him on the street while 'His opponents shop at competing stores, sit far away from the Allands in church, and avoid them on the street' (Rosenberg, 1988: 199).

The most elaborate set of factions is probably the seventeen in Siena, which confront each other on the *palio*: the religiously symbolic horse race (Dundes and Falassi, 1975; Park, 1992) run twice a year. The seventeen factions – *contrade* – are based in the seventeen wards of the city, and Sienese inherit a membership and fierce loyalty to their *contrada*. Each of the seventeen has a flag, a patron saint, a chapel, a treasury and a 'government'. When babies were born at home, families made sure they were delivered in the 'correct' *contrada*: now the bed in the maternity hospital has a tray of soil from the *contrada* underneath it so the baby is delivered on the earth of the family's *contrada* (or the flag of the *contrada* will do). In the *palio* ten of the seventeen *contrada* have a representative horse, and the winner is the whole *contrada*, not just the horse and rider. Children grow up with loyalties and hostilities: if your own faction cannot win, then whoever defeats your 'enemy' gets your support.

Religious factionalism can also have political consequences. Bax (1983a: 167) has discussed how Elschberg, a 'small, ordinary village' had become divided between the followers of local monasteries who offered a pre-Vatican II style of Catholicism with saints, processions and statues, and followers of the parish priest who preferred a more 'modern' austere Catholicism. This religious division carried over into 'political' politics in the village. In another small town, Roersel, a similar division had occurred (Bax, 1985b). To understand politics in that area of The Netherlands, it is necessary to grasp the impact of Vatican II on Catholics, and the increasing gap between 'supporters' and opponents.

The most extreme type of factionalism is the vendetta, where opposing groups actually kill each other. Makris (1992) is an acount of researching vendetta in Crete, and the scholars of Sicily and Sardinia have also focused on them. Because such feuding is illegal, it is hard to study and is not discussed further here, except to emphasise that within living memory many communities 'solved' their faction fights by killing.

LOCAL PATRONAGE

Anthropologists in Europe have been particularly interested in patronage, and patron–client relationships. Since Pitt-Rivers (1954) studied Alcala, researchers have returned from Mediterranean cultures with stories of patrons and clients, some admiring the skills of the peasant in using his or her patrons; others bewailing the clientelist politics and blaming them for the backwardness of undeveloped regions.

The idea of patronage is that peasants who need to deal with forces outside their village – such as the state bureaucracy to get a driving licence – will seek a person with more wealth, education, social status or 'pull' to intercede on their behalf. They give their intermediary deference, loyalty, support in village politics and, perhaps, presents of farm produce. The patron gathers a following of clients, which provides him (or her, although most of the studies deal with men) with status, votes in local political contests and the 'buzz' which comes from being a successful 'fixer'. Galt (1974: 182) summarises this:

> The institution of patronage is seen as a way for the peasant to cope with the impersonal, unfair and often hostile demands emanating from national and regional centres to the rural hinterlands.

Rogers (1991: 110) makes a similar point about Ste Foy:

> In their sharply hierarchical view of the world, Ste Foyans see themselves, both individually and collectively, near the bottom of the pecking order, and believe that the only fruitful manner of making their way is to maintain avenues of contact with well-positioned persons (*pistons*). Most are highly skilled in the art of *pistonnage*; believing that impersonal, formal channels are virtually useless, their response to a wide range of difficulties and opportunities is to think of someone who knows someone in a position to pull a string.

Rogers illustrates this with a story about going to Lourdes with a villager, Mrs Verdier. Rogers thought that because it was not the middle of the pilgrimage/tourist season, they would get a hotel room on arrival with ease. Mrs Verdier was equally sure they would be cheated or end up with nowhere to sleep unless they used *pistonnage*. Mrs Verdier therefore asked a farm labourer in Ste Foy for the name of a hotel in Lourdes where his sister worked as a maid, and when they got to Lourdes sent Rogers to find the sister, to get them a room either in 'her' hotel or an equivalent one where the sister would have a contact. Rogers, being American, found this too embarrassing, and went to the hotel and booked a room at reception. She merely asked to see the Ste Foy maid to send her family messages. Mrs Verdier was happy that her networking had achieved them a room, Rogers had not been embarrassed but recognised that 'it is possible that I also disrupted some elaborate exchange of favours' (1991: 110).

In Seville the term for patrons is *enchufes* (literally electric plugs) or *cuna* (door stops, a person who holds the door open for you), and Press (1979: 98) comments: 'Only the foolish or unconnected allow government or bureaucratic procedure to dominate them unchallenged.'

A typical example of a peasant population dependent on patronage for help with bureaucrats outside the village, comes from an ethnography of Portugal, although it is an example where *women* have the family's patronage ties, rather than men. Riegel-haupt (1967) studied a village, São João das Lampas, some 40 kilometres from Lisbon. There were 363 people living there when she conducted her fieldwork in 1962. Politics was largely a matter of using contacts (*conhecimentos*), and it was women who had more chance to make links to people who can act as contacts. Women made contacts either through domestic service or selling rural produce. Many of the women from São João had been servants in urban, middle- or upper-class families before marriage (when they returned to the village). Contacts would be maintained with employers, who could help in dealings with bureaucrats. Women also travelled (on donkeys) to Lisbon or a nearby town to sell fresh vegetables and bread to regular customers. Such customers could also be enlisted as *conhecimentos*. Men rarely travelled outside São João, and had no chance to establish regular commercial or close domestic links to middle- or upper-class urbanites. This was Portugal under the Salazar dictatorship, and inside villages the priest was often the only literate person, and therefore an import-ant link to government. By the time O'Neill (1987), Pina-Cabral (1986) and Brettell (1986) came to study rural Portugal, the patterns of patronage had changed somewhat. In particular, the importance of the priest as a patron had declined.

Galt (1974: 185) found that on the tiny island of Pantelleria the inhabitants believed they needed a patron: 'to change a large denomination [banknote]' and even more so to deal with 'the commune, the banks, the post office, the employment office, and the airlines office'. If an islander crossed to Sicily or to the main-land 'friends' became even more vital. So on Sicily, as in mainland Italy, patronage links are considered necessary to deal with almost everything including: 'hospitals, police officers, universities, regional government offices, and the civil service system' (p. 185).

Galt quotes one informant describing how his government com-pensation for flood damage had not arrived, although he had done all the paperwork. The informant went to the Agricultural Inspector's office and found someone who knew a man called Giovanni who came from his village on Pantellaria. That official found his file, and he got his money but: 'my aunt, who has lands in the same area, who was visited by the same engineer, and had the same amount of money coming . . . she is still waiting' (p. 189). Galt (1974) asked his informant and his field assistant why recommendations (*raccomandazioni*) are needed to get a form processed, and the field assistant explained that all the papers lie in heaps, and people with 'pull' get their papers queue-jumped, leaving the files of those without influence to slide further and further down the piles. Galt comments: 'A glance at the bank in Pantelleria . . . reveals dog-eared bundles of records haphazardly stacked in open cabinets and shelves' (p. 190). Galt, an American, is clearly shocked when he writes that:

> even the simplest act of drawing money out of a savings account in the bank on the island takes forty-five minutes to an hour, and the form one fills out passes through the hands of three people.
>
> (p. 192)

Getting action on a file from a government office takes much longer. There is even a poetic phrase for such files they are said 'to be *in giacenza*' which has connotations 'of a corpse lying in a tomb' (p. 190). Sensible people in Pantelleria cultivate relationships with doctors, school teachers, civil servants, officers of the carabinieri (a type of police force), those in local government and even caretakers in the buildings of bureaucracies. The sensible person is *furbo* – crafty, streetwise, a wheeler-dealer – a person who uses contacts and networks to get a response from the inefficient bureaucracy. Only a fool – *fesso* – waits for justice to come to him unaided. A man's status is partially based on his manipulation of his 'strong friends'.

An outsider might wonder what the patron gets out of providing favours for clients. If the 'patron' is a low-paid official, then gifts of grapes, a chicken, a few eggs, a fresh lettuce, are not to be sneezed at. Galt describes the power held by low grade 'porters' at Palermo university over students, and points out that the gifts they get are an important supplement to their pay. The client can offer a variety of things, even if he is very poor he can provide something: 'He could collect mushrooms, raise rabbits as gifts, act as a spy and even (as is the case in mafia networks) commit murder' (1974: 187).

All clients also have one valuable 'gift': their votes. Many patrons want votes. The mayor, the local councillors, the delegates to regional assemblies, the member of the national parliament, even the minor judiciary need to be elected into office. If they can fix something, they can get a vote. It is at this point that local patron–client politics meet national politics, the topic of the next section. Before that topic, however, some further examples of patronage in areas less desolate, isolated and peripheral than Pantelleria are provided. France is a more 'modern' society than southern Italy, but patronage is just as vital. Rosenberg (1988: 195) for example says: 'Patronage has been the dominant idiom of political life in the Hautes-Alpes since the mid-nineteenth century.'

Although Abriès is a long way from Paris, it is important because French political careers are built on a local base. The Hautes-Alpes is a region of career building.

> A neophyte politician is 'parachuted' into a local political arena, is elected on the promise of bringing some economic benefit to the locality, and may hope to move on to higher public office eventually.
>
> (1988: 195)

Peasants in regions like the Hautes-Alpes are so dependent on subsidies that their votes are only 'useful' if 'sold' to a patron. The locals called their strategy 'peasant diplomacy', but Rosenberg thinks this a euphemism: 'Peasant diplomacy in practice means exchanging votes for subsidies and supporting with a long reach (and "big sleeves") who can penetrate the system and get access to money' (p. 196). One very conservative villager said: 'I'd vote for a communist if he had good connections' (p. 196) which meant someone with '*personnalité*'. In local affairs, a former mayor, Jean Alland and the former village secretary, Madame Belier, are useful patrons. Madame Belier is used to sort out pensions, and people 'repay' her by being deferential to her, 'accompanying her to church or choir practice' and by patronising her nephew's grocery shop. This is typical of how a local patron is rewarded.

In Ste Foy the lowest tier of elected office is a fifteen-member town council. Rogers (1991) argues that membership of that town council gives access to higher level, more powerful contacts beyond Ste Foy. Thus, from the viewpoint of low-status people in Ste Foy, it is sensible to vote onto the town council high-status people who will have good contacts, make good contacts, and defend the interests of Ste Foy. In 1976 a candidate stood on a platform of being 'of the people', and untainted by 'power or privilege' (p. 112). The locals thought these were exactly the reasons he should *not* be elected. His opponent was a friend of the mayor and of the Archbishop of Paris – he got elected.

Much of the research on patronage has been done in Italy, including a comparison of two towns Luco and Trasacco in the Abruzzio, central Italy, by White (1980). She was fiercely hostile to the patron–client system pointing out that:

> the phrase that is used . . . *scambio di favori* (exchange of favours) [gives] clientelism legitimacy . . . Scarce resources such as jobs, loans, grants, electrical and water connections, tarred roads and so forth are distributed (or often only promised) in exchange for political support. The 'client' gives his own vote and his energy in recruiting the votes of others for the party of his benefactor. But the exchange is not an equal one, despite the language used to describe it.
>
> (1980: 5)

White argues that the patron distributes or withholds the means of subsistence and a decent standard of living, while the client gives up his class interest and rights to class struggle.

White set out to study the Fucino area, where most of the *comuni* support the Christian Democrat party and are riddled with clientelist politics, but there was also Luco, a Communist stronghold where the population regarded clientelism as 'backward, immoral and degrading' (1980: 5–6). She chose Trasacco as the village where she could study clientelism, which would contrast with Luco.

Trasacco had 5,311 residents in 1971, most of whom lived in the village and went out from it to farm. The land was very fertile, and there was also a paper mill and some small factories. Desirable jobs, such as school teaching or the post office are in short supply. A teaching post gets 200 applications, and there is also a surplus of doctors. White describes the key patrons in Trasacco. The parish priest, Don Pasquale, is needed to give *raccomandazioni* if women want to to work at the shirt factory. Dr Ciofani, the commune doctor: 'controls so many things: jobs in the factories, beds in the hospital, places in the football team, you name it' (p. 56). White was told it was believed that Dr Ciofani controlled which doctors got appointments at the state hospital in Avezzano, and the jobs at the electronics factory. The villagers actually thought Ciofani was an incompetent doctor and his surgery was usually empty, but they kept their official registrations with him because of his power. When they were ill, they saw Dr Dalla Monta, even if they had to queue from 7 a.m. to 12 noon to see him. Many women in Trasacco told White that they would vote for anyone who would help their

husband in the post office get transferred to Trasacco; for anyone
who got their son a job; for the person who could get their
children into the right classes at their schools; or to get themselves
a job.

White describes a community where there is fear, distrust and
hypocrisy. People are scared to get onto the wrong side of the
patrons, so hide their real views.

> A student complained that because he was known in Trasacco as a
> communist, a fellow student, his closest friend in Rome, would not
> give him so much as a flicker of recognition in Trasacco.
>
> (1980: 58)

Similarly two medical students who were left-wing at university
always talked like Christian Democrats in Trasacco to keep in with
Dr Ciofano. The clientelist politics of Trasacco does not deliver
efficient municipal services: much of the village was unpaved and
the commune was in debt. White is clear that the clientelist politics
are to blame for the demoralisation of the population and the
poor state of the village. Trasacco sounds like Montegrano and
many other towns and villages of the Italian south. White's other
research site, Luco, was very different.

Luco had 4,610 residents in 1970 and is only 7 kilometres away
from Trasacco, but as White describes it, life there is very different.
Luchesi get more out of their farm land, partly because they have
invested in machinery and women work in the fields. Farming
skills are valued, so that at the 1970 festival for the Madonna a
tractor gymkhana was a highlight. Manual work was not despised,
but regarded as honourable, whether in the factories or on the
land. The biggest difference was the absence of fear and clientelism. In Luco politics was a matter of open membership of either
the Christian Democrats or the Communists, not selling votes for
promises of jobs or hospital beds.

White discovered that neither the doctors nor the priests had
built up clients in Luco, and while the priest tried to get people to
vote Christian Democrat he did so publicly as a matter of political
principle, not by personal favours and threats. *Luchesi* told White
that they 'will not stand for clientelist practices' (1980: 124).
Stories were told of angry refusals to vote for a man called Biagino
Venditti who wanted to trade votes for (much prized) jobs in the
state forestry's tree nurseries. People suspected of using politics for
personal gain were called *ruffiani* (a terrible insult which means a

pimp). Overall Luco was 'an "open" place, both socially and politically' (p. 159). A lawyer from Milan told White that: 'The *luchesi* farm with their brains, the *trasaccani* send their brains to university' (p. 159).

For White clientelist politics was one result of inequalities of land tenure and access to jobs, but also a barrier to tackling those problems. Some social scientists have written about patronage as, if not a good system, one which at least gives poor people some power and a decision-making role. Galt, White and Rosenberg all emphasise that patronage is a vicious circle. Because each individual is reduced to using personal favours and negotiating skills to manipulate the system, the poor and powerless have no motivation to bond together and campaign to get the system to work equitably, even if such bonding together were legal (and in much of Europe it has not been legal for long periods of this century). That course is a long haul, with no certainty of success, while asking your aunt's employer's brother to move your file up the heap is certain to solve your problem. The more powerful people, who have more chance of changing the system, have no motivation to do so either, for their status is based on being 'fixers'. The clients cannot risk trying to change the system, and the patrons have no motivation to do so. There are also scholars who object to the whole tone of the debates on clientelism, arguing that *all* human life is based on networks and calling in of favours, and that an author like Galt is condemning in Pantelleria the same system that he operates himself to get his doctoral students jobs, his friends on to committees, get grants for his colleagues and so on. Boissevain (1974) has argued that *all* human societies run on patron–client networks, and the researchers who disapprove of them in southern Europe are blind to them in their own lives. Certainly a society where 'the old boy network' and 'the old school tie' are seen as ways to get ahead cannot really claim to be free of clientelism.

White's preference for the sturdy independence of the people in Luco, and her pity for the patronage-ridden Trasacco, are explicit. She is confident that the lives of peasants are better when politics is an open matter of contest between national parties. Her enthusiasm for Luco, with its open contest between the two major parties, leads on to the next theme of the chapter, national politics and local issues.

NATIONAL POLITICS AND LOCAL ISSUES

One of the most readable and accessible studies of the interface of national and local politics is Kertzer's (1980, 1990) work on Bologna. Kertzer, an American, was concerned to answer what: 'to most Americans . . . is a great mystery' namely 'the strength of the Italian Communist Party (PCI)' (1990: xv). In 1979, for example, a third of all the votes cast in Italy were for the PCI, although Italy is still a strongly Roman Catholic country and the Church is resolutely opposed to Communism in the world and the PCI in Italy. So in 1971 Kertzer went to live in Albora, a *quartiere* of Bologna outside the city walls, where 9,000 working-class Italians lived, two-thirds of them voting for the PCI in elections.

Kertzer shows that in this neighbourhood there were two political systems. A person was either active in the Catholic Church and the Christian Democrat Party (DC) *or* in the Communist Party (PCI). There were parallel systems of patronage: people either used the priest to get them jobs, flats and hospital beds *or* an official in the PCI. The few men who were active Catholic laymen (for here as in much of Catholic Europe, women make up the bulk of churchgoers) were employed in government jobs, or in banks or companies run by leading DC activists or in Catholic hospitals.

The Italian Catholic Church, like the Maltese, has been vehemently anti-Communist for many years and the DC party shares this perspective. Pratt (1984) is an analysis of DC posters and rhetoric in the post-war period, which shows how Catholicism, 'family values' and voting DC are depicted as three intertwined bulwarks against Soviet tanks (i.e. the PCI). In Bologna the main result of this attitude is to reinforce the majority of the population's adherence to the PCI. In Albora people used the church for marriages and funerals, send their children for catechism classes, but do not regularly attend mass, and shut their ears to the anti-PCI propaganda. Residents of Albora did not antagonise the priest, because it was always possible a *raccomandazione* from a priest will be needed, but their primary allegiance was to the PCI.

That fieldwork was completed in 1972, but Kertzer returned to Albora in 1990. In the interim the DC had held their national position, but the PCI had undergone various crises, and a non-Communist but anti-DC party, the Socialists led by Craxi, had risen in national importance. In Albora the DC had lost ground, but so too had the PCI, partly because public, communal, street life had declined in favour of domestic privacy. One of the two priests, Don Luigi, was still alive and at work in Albora.

> Today, Don Luigi lamented, people's religion is neither that of the Church nor that of the Communists, but of consumerism . . . He no longer sees the PCI as the primary enemy of the Church in the parish; rather it is consumerism and the privatisation that goes with it. At least the Communists thought about the Church, if only to oppose it. Today, sighs Don Luigi, most people don't even think about the Church.
>
> (Kertzer, 1990: 286)

Abeles (1991) is a parallel study in France to Kertzer's work in Italy. Abeles immersed himself in the department of Yonne, 'the provincial heartland of France' (p. xvii). He studied Quarré-les-Tombes a rural mountain area, wine-growing areas, and the industrial centres, plus the chief town. Auxerre, on the banks of the Yonne has a population of 42,000 and was Abeles' choice as the centre of an anthropological study of French politics. Abeles used real names, because his characters are politicians whose lives are already in the public domain. Because in the French system: 'it appears to be almost impossible to achieve national prominence without first having served your time as a town councillor, mayor, or member of the General Council' (p. xviii). Abeles felt that local politics was of national interest. Except at election times, politics are of little interest to the people of Yonne, but Abeles contrasts this lack of enthusiasm among the majority with the commitment of the few active politicians.

In Quarré-les-Tombes Abeles studied the 1983 elections for the municipal council. The outgoing mayor and his faction were mostly re-elected, while an opposition group mostly failed except for one retired schoolmaster who was known as a 'decent' man although left wing. Also elected was an Independent called Truchot, who did not seem to have any experience or any policies. Abeles was amazed: Truchot was only 30, was a farmer and seemed uninterested in politics. Locals told Abeles that Truchot had been elected 'because of his name' (p. 15). It transpired that Truchot was not unknown at all. His grandfather had been mayor, and he was seen as the true heir of a great anti-clerical, radical tradition in the commune. He did not *need* to put forward any policies: his position was taken for granted, and by making no case he gained votes for his modesty. For the locals Truchot was the 'natural' or the 'obvious' (p. 18) choice. When Abeles did historical research he could trace local political dynasties back to 1789 in this region, for it had been divided between anti-clerical radical (red) and conservative (white) groups for 200 years. (The red versus white division is discussed later in this chapter.)

An outsider might think the rural area of Quarré-les-Tombes was a backwater *because* its politics were still patterned on dynasties with local roots. In fact the same deep-rooted *historical* aspect was equally prominent in the town of Auxerre. The continuities in Auxerre politics, despite the growth of the town over the past fifty years, were apparent when Abeles studied the history of the mayors. In the French system the mayor is a very important political figure locally, and being a mayor is an important basis for building a national political career. Auxerre has only had three mayors in seventy years, one of whom was in power for thirty years. Here too memories are long, political dynasties have deep roots, and national politics are less important than a belief in a person who can be trusted to do his best for the town. In one way, national issues (such as a secular or a Catholic education system) *are* important in the Yonne, but only as part of a pattern where long memories colour political choices.

Anthropologists have not done much research on political issues except at the local level, and many of them, like Aschenbrenner (1986) in Karpofora and everyone who worked in Spain, Portugal and Greece while they had dictatorships, has avoided political issues to concentrate on kinship or religion, Loizos's (1975) work on Cyprus being an unusual exception.

The fourth theme of this chapter is that of stratification: who becomes a patron and who is doomed to be a client? Who are the élite and who are the masses? The anthropological work on this issue has been focused on how far social status can be achieved by being an honourable man, even if a poor one, and how far wealth is necessary to be honourable. Thus anthropological discussion has raised the issue: can a poor man be honourable?

STRATIFICATION AND HONOUR

Stratification is a term social scientists borrowed from geology, who use it to describe the way different types of rock are lying in layers, or *strata*. In human societies different types of people are arranged in strata, with the people at the top having more of what society values than those at the bottom. If a society values camels, then those at the top of the heap have more camels than those at the bottom, if it values power then the top people are more powerful, if it values holiness then those at the top are *more* holy than those at the base. Human societies can be stratified by age, by sex, by race, by caste, or by class and wealth. If the principle is age then the oldest people will have most wealth and power, if it is sex then men rule women, if it is race then all members of one race are superior to those of others irrespective of the merits of individual members of the race and so on.

Among European anthropologists there are some who argue that the village or neighbourhood they studied was egalitarian, others who found highly stratified communities, and many who disputed the findings of others. Inequalities of wealth and status and how to interpret them have provoked some of the most heated debates in anthropology. The topic is also complicated because there may be genuine differences in actual wealth and poverty, in how inequalities are understood and in how anthropologists have studied the topic between one region and another, or even between one community and another. White (1980), for example, argues that Luco and Trasacco have different stratification systems and they are only 7 kilometres apart. There does seem to be a difference between the Mediterranean parts of Portugal, Spain and France and southern Italy and Greece where a man's status *does* seem to be related to the respectability of 'his' women, especially in the working and middle classes, and northern Europe where the status of a man is more dependent on his own behaviour and possessions than on the virginity of his daughters and the faithfulness of his wife.

In this section, the debate about honour and wealth in southern Europe is examined first, before the material on the northern 'half' of the continent. Many anthropologists of the Mediterranean have argued, following Pitt-Rivers (1977), that around that inland sea social status is dependent on a man's honour (or the honour of 'his' women) rather than his wealth. Others, especially Davis (1977), have disputed this vigorously. Pitt-Rivers (1954) began this debate, claiming that in his hamlet, or in Andalusia generally, inequalities of wealth (and of education, political power and jobs) were less important to men than inequalities in honour. So a man who was wealthy, but was too weak to police the behaviour of his daughters and his wife, would have lower status in the village than a poorer man whose daughters were protected virgins and whose wife was a devout, respectable, faithful stay-at-home who aroused no gossip. Subsequently Pitt-Rivers (1977) argued that this was true all round the Mediterranean, and it was one of the region's unifying features.

There are several problems with Pitt-Rivers's original claim, and with his subsequent generalization based upon it. Davis (1977) was particularly critical. Davis agreed that honour is a form of stratification. Not everyone can be equally honourable because it is competitive but he doubted if Pitt-Rivers's villagers were actually indifferent to inequalities of wealth. Davis is suspicious: he suspects that it is easier to be honourable if you are rich. Pitt-Rivers in *People of the Sierra* (1954) claimed that everyone was equal and *all* could be honourable. Davis doubts both, and thinks that very poor men lose honour. Davis is convinced that it is easier for a man to police 'his' women if he is wealthy: they do not need to do agricultural work, or work for outsiders, they can even be chaperoned by servants. A man whose daughters will inherit wealth can vet their suitors more stringently and so on. The issue of honour and shame and relations between the sexes is the focus of Chapter 9, and is not elaborated further here, but it is important to realise that in southern Europe a man who was a cuckold would not be considered manly enough for political office, whereas a man with a mistress would have gained status at the expense of the father/brother/husband of his mistress. Here the emphasis is on inequalities of wealth and how these relate to politics.

However, it is not possible to distinguish totally between political and sexual stratification. Machin (1983: 108) explains:

> Reputation, which rests on the readiness of men to act in defence of their families and on the virginity, chastity and demeanour of related women, is treated as though it were a scarce resource, a material rather than an immaterial commodity. Indeed, since one's reputation may determine whom one marries, it is very much a material concern.

That is, the reputation of a man as a guardian of female chastity is partially a financial matter, and also partially political.

One problem facing researchers is that most villagers tell 'their' anthropologist that their village has no leaders, no-one is superior to anyone else, and the only problems are gossip and envy, not leaders. Almost all the studies of southern Europe report that 'their' community is strenuously egalitarian but researchers have to treat such claims with scepticism. It is true that peasants *tell* outsiders, especially researchers, that their village or hamlet or neighbourhood is made up of equals, but this may not be true if you actually look at resources. This claim to equality is commoner in southern Europe, but not restricted to the south. The community studies done in Wales (e.g. Rees, 1950) claimed that there were no class inequalities in rural Wales, except those imported by the English. O'Neill (1987) who studied a tiny hamlet in northern Portugal tries vigorous demolition of the 'egalitarian' idea. He says the people in his hamlet did not even claim to be egalitarian. So if there is an idea that everyone *is* equal, it may not apply in 'northern' Europe, and 'northern' starts halfway 'up' Portugal.

If we start with those communities close to the Mediterranean where researchers have been *told* that the village is an egalitarian one, we need to know whether it is 'true', and why anthropologists have believed it. One reason for anthropologists arguing that in 'their' village everyone is equal is partly because the richest people, such as the absentee large landowners, are rarely 'locals' and do not appear in the studies. As Bailey (1971b, 1971c) points out in a village 'everyone is equal' because they are all powerless up against the power of the centre: the capital; the rich; the government; the bureaucracy; and the church.

Most communities *claim* to researchers that everyone is equal, or that they were in the past before tourism or some other evil changed everything. They may believe it, or they may be asserting a value: telling the outsider what a good community they are, or they may be expressing Bailey's (1971a) point that compared to rich city folk (or educated anthropologists) they are all equally poor and powerless.

It is often difficult for a researcher to test claims of equality. People are likely to hide their wealth from outsiders, and be suspicious of those who want to count catches of fish landed or flocks of sheep, or measure yields of grain. Official records may be inaccurate because sensible peasants lie to bureaucrats. It has been possible for some researchers to gather detailed data on inequalities of land ownership, and Davis (1977: 81–89) compares wealth and landowning in five studies. It is clear that in most communities where wealth can be or has been measured, there are inequalities. These may or may not be recognised by the locals, and may or may not be reported to researchers. It is also the case that most studies report changes in wealth and class stemming from tourism or industrialisation or agricultural change. So in many communities some groups may be getting wealth from novel sources, although often the old élite are best placed to benefit from new developments.

Status in a community may not be dependent on wealth, although patrons are usually among the wealthier people in a community. Status is partly dependent on respectability and maintaining local standards of family life. High status often rests on living in civilised places and in a civilised manner. In southern Europe that often meant in a town rather than on the farm land, even when that led to inefficient use of time getting to and from the plots. In Ronda (Corbin and Corbin, 1987) being overlooked by your neighbours maintained honour, that is a family was honourable if the visitors who come and go are respectable, and the family's own comings and goings are clearly for good purposes: church, work, school, college. Country living was suspect because it was not public in the same way.

In many cultures city or town life is believed to be higher status than country life, so white-collar jobs have higher status than manual ones because they are done in town. This explains the higher status of white-collar jobs in many societies. Both in Friedl's (1962) village of Vasilika and in Juliet du Boulay's (1974) village Ambeli, families try to marry daughters out of the village to men with jobs in the city or at least in a town.

Education may be a source of status. Loizos (1975) and Boissevain (1965) both report that education is a source of honour and status in a Cypriot and a Maltese village respectively. For Italy it is clear from White's (1980) *Patrons and Partisans* how important education can be, for in Trasacco parents made strenuous attempts to get sons educated and off the land. Loizos (1975) reports a triumphal song sung by a bride's mother: 'I've had six children and they're all educated' (Davis, 1977: 186). Here a woman was boasting about the status of her family, whose respectability is proved by the six educated children. Similar themes turn up in the mourning songs of the Mani (Seremetakis, 1991) discussed in Chapter 10. Having an education can be a way to gather clients, especially when levels of literacy are low, and lots of clients means honour and status. Priests were often important patrons, because they were educated.

If there are differences in wealth (and education and power) in a community, the relations between rich and poor may be more or less hostile. Pitt-Rivers (1954) argued that patron–client ties, which he interpreted benevolently, bound rich and poor together in Alcala. Gilmore (1980) found no such cross-class links in Fuenmayor: indeed he found nothing but hostility and a gaping void between rich and poor there. Reading Gilmore's bleak portrayal of Fuenmayor it is hard to reconcile with Pitt-Rivers's warm account of Alcala. Brandes (1992) who has done research both in Andalusia and in Castile found class inequalities more marked and more hostile in Andalusia, and the debate will no doubt continue for many years to come.

Corbin (1979) provides a brief account of the class system on Ronda, which had 17,000 inhabitants in the 1960s. At the top of the hierarchy are three categories of 'the wealthy and well-educated' (p. 104), two locally grounded and one outsiders. One local top group are the large landowners (señoritos). These families own more than 200 hectares and do not have to do the manual work themselves. The workers on these farms are usually employed for life, and have a bond over and above the simple one of boss/worker, because of their long association with the same estate. The second group of well-educated and wealthy are the commercial and financial 'class', who had made money in the past thirty years from banking, property and factories. They are richer than the señoritos, but less self-confident. The 'outsider' wealthy are professionals from elsewhere in Spain, who are not part of local society. Below the weathy and educated are a mixture of people: 'artisans, shopkeepers, truckers, salesbrokers, clerks and small farmers' (p. 107). Then comes the majority of the population, the workers. In the the town are 'masons, carpenters, painters, plumbers and electricians' (p. 107) and the remaining farm labourers who own a little land themselves. Below them are the day-labourers, and beyond the 'normal' society, the gypsies. Corbin (1979) argues that in Ronda there was no sign of the patronage ties Pitt-Rivers found in Alcala cross-cutting and mitigating class inequalities, but rather the hostilities reported by Gilmore (1980).

The anthropology of northern Europe has not focused on patronage, and there has not been the same desire to deny inequalities of wealth. Writers on Wales have claimed that class distinctions were imposed by the English, and the studies of the west coast of Ireland and the Scottish islands have focused on the poor, but there has not been the same emphasis on egalitarianism that Pitt-Rivers made for southern Spain. In the north of Europe, politics has often been a matter of religious divisions, between Catholics and Protestants, the subject of the next section.

POLITICS AND RELIGION

In many parts of Europe politics is inextricably linked with religion. Traditionally in Wales, for example, Anglicans voted conservative and Nonconformists voted liberal. In Northern Ireland Protestants are Unionists and Catholics are not. In England political allegiance is not popularly associated with religious belief, so it is particularly hard to understand the passions of Northern Ireland, and to recognise in other European countries that '*Christian* Democrats' are an important political force.

Politics and religion are inextricably linked in Northern Ireland, and were so linked in Wales. In the northern countries the main way religion and politics intersect is through Catholicism versus Protestantism, in the southern countries, between Communism and religion. Larsen (1982a, 1982b) is an ethnographic account of how Catholics and Protestants are divided in the political and social life of a town, Kilbroney, in Northern Ireland. In Italy and in Malta Boissevain (1965) and Kertzer (1990) both analyse the inter-relationships between the Catholic Church and political activity, including the impact of the Catholic Church's campaigns against Communism, including refusal of church funerals to Communists and even threats of excommunication. In France many rural areas saw conflict between the 'red' and the 'white' factions, where the 'whites' are the equivalent of the DC supporters in Italy, wanting Catholic values to suffuse politics, education and social policy. The 'reds' want a separation of church and state, so that an individual's schooling is secular and their Catholicism, if any, is a private matter. Morin (1971: 177–178) is an account of the struggle for control of the schooling of Plodemet's children between the reds and the whites.

The final theme of this chapter is one even more remote from the UK: bandits and mafia.

MAFIA AND BANDITS

Much of this chapter has been about Italy, and the last topic which has to be briefly mentioned is a particularly Italian one: mafia and bandits.

It may seem odd to have a section on bandits and mafia in a book on modern Europe, and in the chapter on politics. There is a substantial literature on the topic which is only mentioned here. In 1959 Hobsbawm argued that when wild peripheral regions are first incorporated into nation states, the response of the men in these regions is often to become bandits. Hobsbawm saw this as an heroic working-class response, which would gradually be replaced by conventional trade union and left-wing political activity. Thus banditry was a transitional stage in rural life which 'explained' the outlaws of Sicily and Sardinia. Researchers who have gone into the development of the mafia in Sicily, its equivalent in the toe of Italy, and the Sardinian bandits are sceptical of Hobsbawm's grand theory. Moss (1979) and Blok (1974), dealing with Sardinia and the mafia respectively address this issue. Schweizer (1988) contains a critical response to the Sardinia debate.

CONCLUSIONS

Politics takes many forms in Europe, from patron–client relations in a small village to the 'parachuting' of a presidential hopeful into a rural French area. Reputation, religion and old school ties may be more important than a politician's 'politics'. In most countries politics is still a man's business, and women who enter political life risk insults and humiliation.

SUGGESTED READING/ACTIVITY

Kertzer's (1990) *Comrades and Christians* is an evocation of the great days of the PCI in Bologna, when it provided an alternative to the Church.

Chapter 8

Turned in prayer
Religion, magic, science and the supernatural

To Mecca thou hast turned in prayer with aching heart and eyes
that burn . . .

(Flecker, 1947: 98)

INTRODUCTION

Since the revelation to the Prophet Muhammed on the mountain
near Mecca in 610 AD, there has been struggle between the Christian
cross and the Islamic crescent for mastery over Europe. If the Islamic
armies had taken Vienna in 1683, Europe might all be Muslim today.
If the Crusades had held the Holy Land Islam might be confined to
Saudi Arabia. The legacies of the Crusades, including the attacks by
Catholics on Orthodox believers (the Catholic crusaders sacked Constantinople, the capital of the Greek Orthodox empire in 1204 and
started a 900-year feud between Catholic and Orthodox Churches)
are still influencing life in Europe. The conflicts of Islam and
Christianity, Catholic and Orthodox, Protestant and Catholic, and
the persecution of Jews by Muslims, Catholics and Protestants are all
longstanding 'religious' troubles which still shape European life.
Anyone who doubts the force of religious issues needs only to think
of Northern Ireland and Yugoslavia.

Islam and Christianity are the two major religions that have to
be understood in this chapter – not at the level of academic
theology, but at the level of the simple believer. Anthropologists
call this *practical* religion (Leach, 1968). Alongside these two great
world religions, there are many beliefs in other supernatural or
magical phenomena: the evil eye, vampires, she-devils and witches.
These are found in all parts of Europe, including Great Britain
(see, for example, Luhrmann, 1989).

This chapter focuses on five aspects of Christianity and Islam, and then turns to magic. 'Christianity' is limited to Roman Catholicism and the Greek Orthodox Church; I do not discuss Protestantism or the Orthodox Churches of Russia, Serbia, Armenia and so on, although they have congregations in the cities of Europe where pockets of believers live. There is for example, a Russian Orthodox Cathedral (St Basil's) in Knightsbridge near Harrods. The themes are pilgrimage, saints, the life cycle, spiritual kinship and popular anti-clericalism. This last is a Christian, specifically a Roman Catholic issue, which is not parallelled in Islam, or Protestantism.

I have written about the religious and magical phenomena as if they were real. That is, I have written that 'the Virgin Mary appeared', 'Fray Leopoldo cured', 'the vampire destroyed', 'the evil eye is diagnosed', and 'the Koran is'. This is partly for stylistic reasons – it is clumsy to write 'Devotees of Saint Andrew believe', or 'followers of Islam think' before every statement. But it is also helpful to get into the spirit of the chapter if one accepts that all these religions and magical phenomena are 'true' and 'real' to their believers. Thus, while I do not personally believe that the Virgin Mary appeared at Fatima in 1917, or in Tinos in 1823, that there are vampires stalking rural Greece, that the Hamadshas' dancing would cure my migraines or that I have a duty to make a pilgrimage to Mecca, understanding Europe involves grasping that millions of people *do* believe those things. So this chapter treats the existence of witchcraft in rural France as a 'social fact' exactly like the EEC milk quotas or the reunification of Germany.

Islam gets less space than Christianity because most of the anthropological research on popular religion *in Europe* has been on Christianity rather than Islam (Gerholm and Lithman, 1988, is one exception to that generalisation). Protestantism has received less attention than Catholicism and Greek Orthodox belief, and there is relatively little here on the practical religion of Protestants in Europe. However it is important for anyone living or studying in modern Europe to understand Islam, because there are Muslim minorities in most countries.

RELIGIOUS BELIEF AND PRACTICE

Pilgrimage

Pilgrimage is an important part of Roman Catholicism and Greek Orthodox life, and is a central part of Islam. One of the duties of a devout Muslim is the *Hadj*: the pilgrimage to Mecca and Medina. There are two kinds of pilgrimage, those to famous shrines, such as Mecca for Muslims, Lourdes for Catholics and Tinos for Greek Orthodox believers, and 'local' pilgrimages to small shrines known only in their neighbourhood, such as that on Nisos (Kenna, 1990). In this section both types of Christian pilgrimage are discussed first, then both types of Islamic pilgrimage.

Turner and Turner (1978) wrote the first serious anthropological work on Christian pilgrimage. Pilgrimage sites grow up from groups of people believing in a *sign* of supernatural intervention in human affairs, and wanting to go to the place where that *sign* appeared. The sign is sometimes an apparition (Fatima, Lourdes, Medjugorje), sometimes a miraculous cure (Padre Pío), and the place where this happened 'vibrates' with religious power/ efficacy. Devotees hope that something miraculous may happen again, and believe that it will do so, if not for them, for others. Pilgrimage sites usually have a story: the tale of the original event that led to the place being venerated, and internationally renowned pilgrimage sites become economically developed as facilities for the devotees are provided. In this discussion stories attached to some sites are retold, with their 'political' significance if any, and their economic consequences set out. The motives of pilgrims are explored after the accounts of local pilgrimages, because the goals of the devotees are essentially similar whether one leaves Liverpool on a five-day bus trip to Lourdes (Dahlberg, 1991) or merely walks a mile along the beach of a Greek island to a local shrine.

France has seen a series of Marian appearances – that is visions of the Virgin Mary – at what later became pilgrimage sites. These include La Salette in 1846, Lourdes in 1858, Pontmain in 1871 and Pellevoisin in 1876. At La Salette (near Grenoble) the Virgin appeared to two illiterate shepherd children. It became a focus for anti-papal groups and is not very fashionable today. The most popular Marian pilgrimage site in France is Lourdes. Bernadette Soubirous, again an illiterate shepherd, saw the Virgin Mary in 1858. The Virgin said she wanted a chapel built on that site outside the village and people to come to it, and also said she was 'the Immaculate Conception', ('*Que soy era Immaculade Councepcíon*') speaking to Bernadette in her Bigourdian dialect, not in French.

Cynics said this claim was very convenient for Pope Pius IX who had made his declaration of the Virgin's immaculate conception three years earlier. Bernadette became a nun, died in a convent which is itself a pilgrimage site now, and was herself canonised in 1933. The hierarchy of the Roman Catholic Church has been supportive of Lourdes, and recognised it as a genuinely religious phenomenon in 1866 when the local bishop invited the Garaison Fathers to take charge of the ceremonies (Eade, 1991).

Lourdes has boomed as a pilgrimage centre since 1858. The town then had a population of 4,000, by 1928 it had grown to 8,000, and by 1980 to 18,000 (Marnham, 1980) with 402 hotels containing 32,000 beds. The pilgrimage traffic led to the railway being extended to Lourdes in the last century, and to an airport in the twentieth. In 1978 486,000 visitors arrived by rail and another 318,000 by air. In 1950 there were an estimated 1.6 million visitors, in 1958 (the centenary) 5 million, in 1970 3.5 million and in 1990 4 million (Dahlberg, 1991). In 1981 the Pope visited the site, and there have been sixty-four 'miraculous' cures attested plus 5,000 others claimed.

Lourdes can be compared with one of the major pilgrimages for Greek Orthodox believers: to Tinos, the home of a famous miracle-working icon, housed in the Church of the Madonna of the Annunciation (*Evangelistria*). Dubisch writes:

> The church draws thousands of pilgrims each year, the majority of them women. These women come to pay their respects to the *Panayia* (the Virgin Mary), to request her help and to fulfil vows. They bring with them all manner of offerings, not the least of which is themselves. Some women walk barefoot all or part of the way to the church, while others crawl the entire distance on their knees, sometimes carrying a child on their backs. They bring candles, flowers, icons, oil, and items they have embroidered or crocheted.
>
> (Dubisch, 1991: 41)

The story behind Tinos is that an icon (the flat paintings of saints, Jesus, Old Testament characters and the Madonna which are the central devotional objects in Greek Orthodox belief) of the mother of Christ (the *Panayia*) had been buried in the debris of a church burned by the Saracens (Muslim pirates) in the Middle Ages. In 1822 the *Panayia* wanted her picture found, so appeared to a nun and told her where it was buried. The local priest organised a half-hearted dig, found nothing and gave up. An epidemic swept Tinos, and people died, so the search for the icon was reinstated and in 1823 it was found. A church was built on the site, completed in 1830 and is the pilgrimage site today.

The years of the vision, 1822/23, were during the Greek War of Independence from their domination by the Ottoman (Turkish) Islamic empire. The church, and independence were both achieved by 1830. Tinos is the most visited shrine in Greece, and the big pilgrimage dates are 15 August (the Assumption or Dormition of the *Panayia*) and 25 March (the Annunciation *and* Greek Independence Day). The actual icon is invisible behind and beneath all the gold and jewels that have been lavished on it. About 200,000 devotees come to Tinos each year, many fulfilling a vow (*tama*) they made to undertake the trip (Dubisch, 1988).

Few of the important Greek pilgrimage sites have been studied by researchers, although they are full of interest. On the island of Rhodes there is a monastery on Mount Tsambika where the icon can help barren women conceive. A supplicant should climb the hill on foot on 8 September, and eat a piece of the wick from a candle from the *Panayia*'s chapel. A baby born after this divine intercession should be called Tsambika or Tsambikos as part of the bargain.

Cyprus too has its Greek Orthodox holy places – and one of the most sacred is now in the Turkish-occupied north of the island – the monastery of Apostolos Andreas. Thubron referred to the site – on a headland – as the 'Lourdes of Cyprus' (1986: 247). St Andreas has worked many miracles, including a family reunion. In 1895 Turkish bandits captured the baby son of Maria Georgiou, and she never thought to see him again. Seventeen years later she dreamt that St Andreas wanted her to come to his monastery and pray for her son's return. On the boat journey to Cyprus she told her story to a young male dervish who turned out to *be* her son, sold into slavery and reared as a Muslim. Before 1974, this was a major Greek pilgrimage site, its current status is peculiar: an Orthodox pilgrimage site marooned in hostile Muslim territory.

Turning back to Roman Catholic pilgrimage sites, the major European ones include Rome itself, to see the Pope and St Peter's, Asissi the home of St Francis, Lourdes and Fatima in Portugal. Children saw the Virgin here in 1917, and she made statements about Russia which believers see being fulfilled with the fall of the Soviet Communist regime. The Republic of Ireland has Knock in County Mayo. In 1879 the Virgin appeared with St John and St Joseph on the wall of the parish church. In 1976 a church which can hold 200,000 opened, and the Pope visited in 1979. The area also got an airport, to bring pilgrims in, due to the political efforts of the local Cardinal, Monsignor Horan.

On Mallorca there is a monastery – Lluc – which houses a tiny, almost black, statue of the Madonna found by a shepherd boy in the twelfth century. This statue (*Nuestra Señora de Lluc*), covered in precious stones and housed behind the high altar of the monastery church, receives thousands of visitors. Devout Mallorquins come on pilgrimage, especially in September, and hundreds of tourists on bus trips also visit *Lamorerata* (The Little Brown One).

Most recently the Virgin appeared at Medjugorje in Yugoslavia – or rather in Hercegovina. This was a remote, unknown mountain village with a population of 3,000 in a predominantly Catholic area, although there are Serbian Orthodox and Islamic minorities in the area. The Virgin appeared to six children here in 1981, and until the Yugoslavian state fell apart and the wars between the ethnic groups began, Medjugorje was building up to be a major pilgrimage site. In the first ten years 15 million pilgrims came to the village (Bax, 1991). National pilgrimage sites are economically significant not only because of the pilgrims but also because of the tourist trade that accrues to them.

Local pilgrimages may be religiously and socially important, for the community that participates. A chapel, cave, shrine or other site associated with a local saint may be visited by people living in the neighbourhood (and any expatriates who return for the festivities) as an outing. Jorion (1982) describes the villagers from Houat going to a shrine of St Anne. Hertz (1913/1983) provides an account of the cult of St Blesse, in the Italian Alps as it was celebrated in 1910/12. Hertz interviewed devotees and collected 'rustic stories' of the 'little saint'. Christian's (1972) work on northern Spain contains material on local pilgrimages.

Sanchis (1983) is a study of Portuguese pilgrimages (*romarias*). He studied 216 pilgrimages in Portugal, mostly rural and not widely known outside their localities. Ninety-nine of the pilgrimage sites were sacred to the Virgin (under sixty-eight different titles), fifty-three to saints, twenty to Christ and fourteen to the Holy Spirit (of which the most famous is at Tomar). Some of the pilgrims Sanchis interviewed were extremely devout and assiduous. One man of 74 was on his thirty-eighth pilgrimage to the shrine of São Bento (Benedict) da Porla Aberta de Geres, a journey of eight hours on foot (p. 267). At the shrine, pilgrims expect to hear sermons which are familiar stories of the saint's life and works. 'What pilgrims want to hear is the Saint's life, repeated to saturation point, and particularly accounts of miraculous episodes which demonstrate his power' (p. 275).

Stories of the miraculous powers of the local saint are equally popular and important to Greek Orthodox pilgrims. Frequently a pamphlet is available (in many languages) retelling the best stories for visitors and pilgrims. The booklet that can be bought in the Orthodox Cathedral of Zakynthos (Zante), by Theoharis Provatakis (n.d.) contains a typical set of such miracles. Saint Dionysios was able to drive out a devil, raise a child from the dead, restore sight to two different blind people, save three drowning sailors, cure a cripple and relieve epilepsy. He also helped several Englishmen, even though they were not Orthodox believers. The *Panayia* icon on Tinos is equally credited with helping not only Orthodox believers, but also with saving the Protestant British consul in a storm at sea, and curing the Ottoman Turkish officer of syphilis (Dubisch, 1988).

Pilgrimages are therefore one important part of Catholic and Orthodox Christians' religious beliefs and practices in Europe. However, going on a pilgrimage is not a duty: a good Catholic does not *have* to go to Fatima, nor is a devout Orthodox Greek in London obliged to go to Tinos unless he or she has vowed to do so. For Muslims, the position is different. The pilgrimage to Mecca is one of the central pillars of the faith (Eickelman, 1976, 1981, 1985; Gilsenan, 1982).

Islam began in 610 AD when Allah sent an angel to Muhammed on a mountain near Mecca, a busy commercial city now in modern Saudi Arabia. This angel revealed Allah's message for the human race – written down in the Koran – and the Prophet Muhammed converted his wife and cousin Ali and began preaching. In 622 he left Mecca for Medina, where he lived till his death in 632.

The Islamic faith has five pillars which are obligations laid on the devout:

1 to profess the faith regularly (the set phrase in English is 'There is no God but Allah and Muhammed is his prophet');
2 fasting from dawn to dusk during the holy month of Ramadan;
3 giving alms to the poor;
4 praying five times a day (facing Mecca);
5 Making the pilgrimage (*Hadj*) to Mecca.

In the days when the *Hadj* was done on horseback, on foot and in sailing vessels, people took months, or even years, to do the journey, many died on the trip and it was a major physical hardship. Roads, railways, steamships and airplanes have put Mecca within the reach of any Muslim who an afford the cost of a trip. About 2 million people now make the pilgrimage each year, from all over the world. Once a person has embarked upon it they are in a 'sacred' state, and if they die go straight to paradise. When pilgrims risked plague, pirates, slave traders, starvation, shipwreck and all the other hazards of a pre-industrial journey it was usual to set off with all one's earthly affairs settled in case of no return. Today people who are old or ill still do that, but younger pilgrims expect to return, although 1,000-2,000 people every year do die on the *Hadj* (Eickelman, 1981).

While in Saudia Arabia a pilgrim will try to visit Medina, where Muhammed died, which is the next most sacred place. Devout Muslims also have other international pilgrimage sites: Kerouan in Tunisia and Cordoba in Spain, which was a centre of Islamic learning and whose mosque still stands 'converted' into a Catholic cathedral. The division between the majority of Muslims (Sunni) and the large sect (Shi'ites) is symbolised by the pilgrimage site of Karbala in modern Iraq, where Hussain, the Prophet Muhammed's grandson, was murdered. Sh'ite Muslims, who believe that Muhammed's nephew and son-in-law Ali was the Prophet's true heir, believe his son Hussain was a martyr, who died gladly so the faithful can enter paradise. Karbala has an annual pilgrimage mourning Hussain's death, when up to a million pilgrims arrive in a town of 30,000 people.

As well as these pilgrimages which are 'officially' part of Islam, there are the equivalents of the local pilgrimages found in Catholic and Greek Orthodox countries. In North Africa especially there are local shrines which are visited by simple people who take offerings and make vows. Many of these shrines are the tombs of holy men, *Marabouts*, who performed miracles in their lifetimes and can do so after their deaths. Theological scholars and educated Muslims reject the whole business of *Marabouts* and their miracles as heresy, but many ordinary people are convinced that going to *Marabouts'* tombs is entirely compatible with being a devout Muslim. There are several studies of such pilgrimages and celebrations at *Marabouts'* tombs in North Africa. Crapanzano (1973) has a vivid account of a ceremony at the tomb of Sheikh al-Kamal in Meknes, Morocco, and also describes the big festival in the village outside Meknes where Sidi Ali is entombed, when pilgrims come from all over Morocco. Rabinow (1977) worked in the city of Sefrou and in a village called Sidi Lahcen which also had the tomb of a powerful *Marabout* to which pilgrims came.

Muslim women do not go to the mosque, although they do go on the *Hadj*, but visits to *Marabouts'* tombs are frequently female affairs. Most of the researchers who have studied women's visits to shrines worked in North Africa. Tapper (1990) reports similar material from Egirdir an agricultural town of 9,000 people in Turkey. Here women from the more traditional families go in all-female groups to shrines on the outskirts of the town, and the petitioner will make a vow there. For women, visits to *Marabouts'* tombs or other shrines are a way of being actively religious *and* having a social event. This exactly parallels the twin functions of pilgrimage in Catholic and Orthodox Christian communities.

Saints

Both the Catholic and Greek Orthodox churches have saints, and there is ample ethnographic evidence that cults of saints are a central part of religious practice. Islamic countries have equivalent figures and although the term 'saint' is used by some scholars to describe them, it carries such Christian connotations that here I have used *Marabout* instead. Again the Catholic and Greek Orthodox material is presented before that on Islam. In this section the Virgin Mary is 'counted' as a saint, because cults of the Virgin, sometimes in a particular manifestation such as 'The Madonna of the Snows' or 'The Star of the Sea' are similar to saints' cults. Believers pray to the Virgin to intercede with God for them, or to a saint to do so.

Wilson (1983a) provides a useful introduction to saints in Catholic and Orthodox Christianity. He points out that saints are controversial figures for theologians. Some are clearly pagan gods adapted – St Anne in Brittany is probably the local Celtic goddess Ana and St Costas and St Damian are the Castor and Pollux of Greek mythology. Others are or may become political – when St Joan was canonised in the pre-1914 era it was a right-wing, nationalist, French campaign that achieved her elevation.

The social structure of saints reflects the social structure of society that venerates them. Saints are mostly *men*, although women are the main supporters of cults. Wilson suggests that cults of the saints are more venerated by poor peasants in marginal areas and the urban poor, than by landowning élites or the bour-geoisie and urban upper classes. In Houat Jorion (1982) found the three important saints were St Anne, the Virgin in her form of *Stella Maris* (Star of the Sea) and St Gildas. Local people make offerings to the Virgin before fishing trips and carry a statue of St Anne or the Virgin on boats.

Wilson's (1983b) own research on the popularity of saints in central Paris neatly measured the faith of ordinary believers. In 1978 during August and September he visited thirty-three churches and seven chapels out of the forty-four in ten districts of central Paris (but not Notre Dame because it is full of tourists not locals.) Wilson then *counted* the statues, the candles and the votive offerings, plus the chapels or altars and the collection boxes that were displayed related to the various devotional figures, such as the Virgin, the various Aspects of Christ and the saints. He found that the most popular devotional objects were: the Virgin Mary, St Theresa, St Anthony of Padua, and the Sacred Heart of Christ. There were thirty-seven statues of the Virgin, while St Theresa, with thirty-two statues, came next.

Saints rise and fall in popularity. Statues are most characteristic of *popular* cults and recent ones. Some nineteenth-century churches have elaborate stained glass windows representing saints no longer popular. For example, in central Paris St Genevieve (patron saint of Paris) was declining in 1978 while St Rita was on the way up. St Rita has a shrine at Ermesinde in Oporto, Portugal which is one of the *romarias* studied by Sanchis (1983). Her cult came from the Iberian peninsula, lived in the fourteenth century, was canonised in 1900 and was 'booming' in central Paris in 1978. Wilson (1983b) found the first offering to her dated from 1968, while there were lots in 1977. That decade had seen a major migration of Spanish and Portuguese women into Paris, and Wilson argues that they were the devotees of St Rita.

'Active' saints have candles lit in front of their statues and female saints may also have flowers. These are different colours for different saints. The Virgin gets white or green or blue flowers while other saints like St Rita get red flowers. Active saints have votive offerings like metal plaques, letters, and so on, attached near them or to them. Most votives are expressions of thanks for exam passes, the birth of a child, improved health, and for surviving the 1914–18 war.

The candles, flowers and votive offerings all indicate that believers are coming to the churches to pray to the saint to intercede with God on their behalf. The cults of saints are the religious equivalent of patron–client relations in politics. Just as the poor person feels too poor and ill-educated to approach the government directly, so too God is believed to be too important to be bothered by requests from ordinary people about driving tests, bad hips, sub-fertility, sick donkeys or a safe return from a fishing trip. A saint or the Virgin Mary will carry the plea to God on the petitioner's behalf.

As well as cults of saints (who have already been canonised) there are cults surrounding figures whose followers are waiting and campaigning for them to *be* canonised. McKevitt (1991a, 1991b) has studied the cult of Padre Pío, a holy man whose followers are campaigning to have his sainthood established. He was born in 1887 in southern Italy, and became a Capuchin friar and then was ordained a priest. From 1916 till his death in 1968 he lived in San Giovanni Rotondo, a town in the mountains of Puglia. In 1918 he was afflicted with the stigmata – the bleeding wounds of the crucified Christ – which remained with him till he died. St Francis of Asissi was the first person to have borne the stigmata which are therefore a sign of extreme holiness. San Giovanni Rotondo became a pilgrimage site, and has grown as a cult centre since Padre Pío died. McKevitt (1991a) argues that Padre Pío combined the roles of mystic, folk healer and official priest, in whom the suffering of Christ was re-enacted. McKevitt (1991b) has studied the devotees of Padre Pío – people who have come to live in San Giovanni Rotondo to be near Padre Pío – and the beliefs of the local people who actually live in the town.

Candace Slater (1990) has collected the stories surrounding Brother Leopoldo de Alparideire, a Capuchin friar who lived from 1864–1956. Brother (Fray) Leopoldo is popular in Granada and that area of Andalusia, and is a parallel figure to Padre Pío, currently not recognised by the Church as a saint. The crypt where he is buried is in a 'sleek new Capuchin church' (p. 3) in Granada, and pilgrims flock to it especially on the ninth of each month because he died on 9 February. Fray Leopoldo was described by a 24-year-old medical student as having a lot of influence with God (p. 15). Literally (*'El enia mucha mano con Dios'*) – he had 'a lot of hand' with God. Christian (1991) is an account of a family turning to Fray Leopoldo. There are at least two other Andalusian candidates for sainthood at present: Conchita Barrecheguren and Andres Manjon who founded the Ave Maria schools for the poor.

Slater had previously collected the stories surrounding Padre
Cicero Romeo Batista, a similar figure in Brazil (Slater, 1986).

These holy men and women being considered for canonisation
by the Catholic Church were real historical figures, but to a
devotee of a saint the 'reality' of the person is not as important as
their power to solve problems, such as ill-health, keeping a child in
the army out of foreign service, conceiving a child or being saved
in a storm at sea. The Breton fisherman who believes that St Anne
saved his life in a storm at sea is not interested in Wilson's (1983a)
suggestion that 'St Anne' is really a Celtic goddess adopted by early
missionaries in Brittany. One of the ways in which the official
theology of the Catholic Church has diverged from the faith of the
ordinary believer was the Second Vatican Council's 'downgrading'
of many saints whose historical reality was considered doubtful by
scholars. To the ordinary believer this was the work of the devil.
(See Bax, 1985b, for an account of dismay felt in the Netherlands
town of Roersel when the clergy downgraded the local saint, St
Gerlach.) The power of a saint may not even depend on him or her
being human. There was for many years in France a cult around
Guinefort, a greyhound, who was believed to be able to heal
children (see Schmitt, 1983).

Saints' cults, and cults around *Marabouts*, can be individual or
communal. In Malta there are societies who raise money throughout the year to have a massive firework display on 'their' saint's
festival day. The bigger the firework display the more the society is
felt to be superior to the followers of other saints in their neighbour. Boissevain's (1965) village was divided between the *partiti* of
St Martin and St Rocco in this way.

In North Africa *Marabouts* have brotherhoods who revere them,
and guard the tomb/shrine. Some of these are very quiet, scholarly
bodies of men, while others go into trances and engage in spectacular
practices like fire eating or snake handling. In Morocco, for example,
the city of Fez contains the tomb of Hmed al-Tijanni, who is the focus
of a brotherhood. Fez is the centre of this brotherhood, where its
central lodge and library are, and is the focus of the brotherhood's
annual pilgrimage. There are subsidiary branches in other Moroccan
towns. The Tijanni brotherhood is a puritanical and pious one, very
different from the ecstatic brotherhood – the Hamadsha – studied by
Crapanzano (1973). Kevin Dwyer (1982: 32) contains an account of a
prayer meeting of the Tijanni – prayers additional to the regular
ritual obligations placed on all Muslims. Crapanzano contains vivid

descriptions of the Hamadsha dancing themselves into a trance. Both brotherhoods call themselves good Muslims, and devout followers of their *Marabout*.

In Catholic countries men form cofraternities, dedicated to a particular saint, which offer masses for the souls of dead members. These have been studied in Malta (Boissevain, 1969: 65) and in Andalusia (Driessen, 1984).

Women are less likely than men to form *communal* organisations to support saints or *Marabouts*, and more likely to visit shrines alone, with kin or women friends. This behaviour is *not* enjoined or even sanctioned by Christian theologians but is a part of many women's lives, whether Catholic, Muslim or Orthodox. It is ironic that in contemporary Lyon the Portuguese woman who believes that the Virgin of Fatima, St Rita and her village patron saint are helping her keep her job, holding off her arthritis and getting her children through their school exams has more in common with her Greek neighbour who believes the *Panayia* of Tinos, St Costas and St Damian and her island patron saint are helping her keep *her* job, warding off *her* arthritis and getting her children through school; *and* with the Moroccan immigrant who believes that Sidi Ali is helping her keep *her* job, warding off *her* arthritis and keeping her children from failing in school, than any one of them does with a scholarly theologian of their 'own' faith.

Islamic immigrants from Turkey or North Africa will have brought their 'popular' Islam with its maraboutism to the EEC countries; and presumably there are brotherhoods now meeting in Berlin and Leuven and Lyon, waiting for anthropologists to study them. Ecstatic maraboutism may well be the next alternative therapy in northern Europe, exactly the way Greek fire walking has 'caught on' in the USA (see Danforth, 1989).

It is no accident that adherents of the same saint or *marabout* form 'brotherhoods'. Religion often impinges onto everyday life through such spiritual kinship, and spiritual kin are often important in patronage networks, the nature of which was outlined in the previous chapter.

Spiritual kinship

One important way in which religious beliefs and practices intersect with everyday life is through spiritual kinship. When, for example, a godparent is chosen, the relationship is one of religious significance as well as political expediency. Du Boulay's (1974) village in Evia, Ambeli, illustrates this. Spiritual kinship, or *Koumbaria*, can begin at the christening or a marriage. The *Koumbaros/a* acts as a wedding sponsor and 'crowns' the couple in the sight of God, or at a baptism puts the oil on the babe which signifies the child's membership of the Christian community. Ideally the *Koumbaros/a* who acts at the baptism should be the wedding sponsor and then the *Koumbaros/a* of the first-born of the marriage, and be bound to the 'godchild' and its family for a lifetime (du Boulay, 1991: 44). Becoming a godparent in Ambeli was an honour, and a sacred act.

Similar relationships are established in Catholicism and in Islam, but are not detailed here. Suffice it to say that a wise parent establishes spiritual kinship ties so the family has a web of connections, legitimated by religion, beyond the family created by blood and marriage.

The next theme in this chapter is the importance of religion for marking the stages of the life cycle. As an individual is born, named, received into his or her spiritual community, marries, and dies, religion is the usual source of the public ceremonies which mark these stages. Sociologists usually talk of status passages (Glaser and Strauss, 1965); anthropologists have been interested in the rituals that accompany them – *rites de passage* – since Van Gennep (1908). Here the focus is on death, but birth, baptism, confirmation and marriage are equally important in Christian cultures, while in Islam the circumcision of boys is an important status passage.

The life cycle and life crises

As well as the life cycle, religion may become particularly important at a time of life crisis, such as a life-threatening illness. Christian (1991) has described an example of this: the case of Lucia. Lucia was a 2-year-old girl from a middle-class family on Tenerife who developed a brain tumour and needed elaborate medical treatment. While the family used all its networks to get excellent medical treatment in Barcelona, a whole range of spiritual and supernatural measures was invoked by neighbours, friends and family. Christian spoke to fifty people who had used religious or magical means to try and help Lucia. First, her parents had Lucia baptised, which they had not bothered to do previously.

Others had special masses said, added Lucia to their regular
prayers, and made promises to specific saints, including the Virgin
who is the patron of the Canaries, Fray Leopoldo and St Rita.
Lucia's uncle vowed to go on a pilgrimage from Tenerife to
Granada to Fray Leopoldo's shrine if the child recovered. When
Lucia recovered he took her to Granada to present her, cured, to
Fray Leopoldo's shrine – thus adding to the power of the cult of
Fray Leopoldo. Religious behaviour and belief may lie dormant
until a life crisis strikes, as it had in much of Lucia's family.
Similarly, events in the life cycle can be triggers to religious activity
– especially death.

Death is the stage of the life cycle where religion is most heavily
involved. There is ethnographic research from Brittany and the
Basque country of France (Ott, 1981; Badone, 1989), Portugal
(Pina-Cabral, 1986), Italy (Pardo, 1989), the Basque country of
Spain (Douglass, 1969), and Greece (du Boulay, 1974; Danforth,
1982; Kenna, 1991a; Seremetakis, 1991).

Important issues among the religious and secular observances
designed to remember the deceased are the idea of a 'good death';
the funeral arrangements; and the care of graves. The care of
graves and other memorials to dead relatives have been studied
particularly in Greece and Portugal. Dead relatives are regarded as
part of a family, and caring for graves is a duty which falls on the
living. Kenna (1976, 1991a) studied such observances, especially
the care of graves, when in Nisos in 1966/67 and again in 1987/88.
She writes:

> One of the themes of the first fieldwork was the relationship
> between the inheritance of property and the carrying out of
> various rituals for the souls of the dead . . . In return for
> property, heirs are obliged to arrange and participate in rituals
> which ensure that the soul of the person from whom the
> property was inherited gets to heaven.
>
> (1991a: 102)

Danforth (1982) has written a whole book on death rituals in
northern Greece, which has extraordinarily evocative
photographs. Seremetakis (1991) deals with death in the Mani,
one of the most desolate and depopulated areas of Greece. Today
many Maniots die away from the Mani, and are returned there for
burial. She writes:

A bus is rented and driven to Mani carrying the urban relatives and the dead in a coffin. Buses full of people are a contemporary sign of death . . . The good death here is the completion of the life cycle, and for a Maniot a good death involves loud, and long lasting, public mourning, with screaming and ritual laments. One reason for returning to the village in the country is that the loud mourning screams are forbidden in city flats.

(1991: 84)

The mourning laments are discussed in more detail in Chapter 10. Here the point is that a proper funeral has to take place in the Mani, in the 'home' village, not in Athens, or Corinth or Kalamata but on one's own soil.

Many European cultures have a clear distinction between a 'good' death and a bad one. Typically, a good death is one that comes peacefully to an old person, who has lived a proper life, left descendants, and their affairs in order, made their peace with God, and is surrounded by family at the end. A bad death is one that comes by violence, or to a young person, or hits before a person has made their peace with God.

Pardo's (1989) account of death and mortuary rituals in inner-city Naples shows how people are concerned to have a 'good death': one which is accepted, and takes place surrounded by close relatives. Pardo studied the poor Neapolitans – the *popolino* – who make clear links between the state of the body and the eventual destiny of the soul. A good death leads to a *buonanima* (a good soul) which leaves the survivors in peace. A good death means:

Certain rules must be observed before death. Close relatives surround the dying person and look after him or her, taking care he or she does not refuse to acknowledge the coming death. A good death depends on such acceptance which, in turn, rests upon a fulfilled life and a quiet dying.

(1989: 107)

A person who refuses to accept their death, or one overtaken by a violent or premature death, may leave a spirit 'hovering forever over that house' (p. 107). The French Basque shepherds studied by Ott (1981) divided deaths into violent ones (*heriotzea*) which included suicide and accidents in the mountains and in the valley; and cold death (*hilhotz*) which is painless, quick and in one's own house. Goldey (1983b: 2) found that in northern Portugal:

dying with good warning, in bed, enabled one to prepare for death with the appropriate, traditional ceremony and do a public accounting – forgiving enemies, blessing friends and children, and paying off one's debts.

It is considered a 'terrible thing' to die away from one's village, or worse, away from Portugal. So:

the dead or dying are brought back to the village for burial . . . there have been instances of dying men being brought back from Lisbon or France or even Canada to die at home.

(1983b: 2)

Goldey stresses how a good death involves kin and neighbours, not only at the deathbed but during the burial and afterwards.

Many cultures have systems where women of the family and neighbourhood deal with the corpse, and it is vital that this is done properly. In those countries where a body is dug up after a couple of years and the bones moved to an ossuary, that too must be properly done if the living survivors are to keep their social status and the dead peoples' souls rest in peace. Du Boulay (1982) has written in detail about the terrible consequences of not burying someone properly – they become an 'undead', a revenant, a vampire (*vrykola*) – one of a class of magical beings discussed in part two of this chapter.

The final theme in this section of the chapter is popular anti-clericalism.

Popular anti-clericalism

The existence of religiosity coupled with anti-clericalism is frequently reported from Catholic areas and by researchers on Greek Orthodox communities about men, especially shepherds. Herzfeld (1990: 309) describes the shepherds of Glendi as: 'in general a cynically anti-clerical group of men'. Men are more frequently reported to be anti-clerical than women, partly because men resent the influence the priest has over women's lives, and partly because priests are not seen as proper men who work for a living, as in Jorion's (1982) study of Houat in Brittany, a fishing community where men face death every time they go out in their boats. The men have an elaborated 'folk' model of Catholic beliefs about death and the after-life. They are anti-clerical but not atheists. Men have contempt for a priest: a man who stays on the land with women and children while 'real men' go out to sea. Women who face death have a priest to mediate with God on their behalf, but men who face death are alone with God at sea. So men equate the priest with feminine weakness, and themselves adopt a robust, unmediated relationship with God.

There are other communities in which popular anti-clericalism is found in both sexes (e.g. Messenger, 1969; Riegelhaupt, 1984). Freeman (1967: 43) argued that the inhabitants of Valdemora, the Castilian hamlet she studied, regarded 'true religiosity' as 'quite separate from the compliance with formal Church dogma'. In 1963 the priest was particularly unpopular and people did not go to confession regularly – indeed 'they expressed real horror at the notion of ever confessing to the present priest'. Instead they confessed to visiting priests, and the rest of the time attended mass but did not take communion. The priest celebrated mass without a pause for communion because he 'knew full well that, without confession, no-one in town was able to receive the sacrament' (p. 43). Religiosity for Valdemorans centred on communal rituals, not individual behaviour.

People may have great faith in a particular saint or saints, go on pilgrimages and make vows, yet be very anti-clerical. In her study of people in Granada who are believers in the sanctity and miraculous powers of Fray Leopoldo, Slater (1990: 81) introduces us to Dolores, a cleaning woman of 27 with an unemployed husband who, although she takes a dim view of institutionalised religion and rarely goes to mass, believes in saints and miracles. Dolores made a vow to Fray Leopoldo for the safe delivery of her first baby. She uses a local healer (curandero) and Fray Leopoldo for solving family problems.

Catholic anti-clericalism has grown since the Second Vatican Council of the early 1960s downgraded or even outlawed many practices central to popular Catholicism. For many European Catholics, the attitude of the clergy to witchcraft, the evil eye, saints' cults, festivals and other 'popular' religious manifestations is alienating. As Favret-Saada (1989: 42) argues:

> the people of the Bocage are conservative in politics as well as in religion. All the farmers are baptized, receive first communion, are buried by the church, and they almost all go to church every Sunday. Yet they are anti-clerical Catholics since they consider most priests to be 'unbelievers'.

Favret-Saada says priests are seen as 'unbelievers' because they do not accept the historical reality of 'local healer saints', or the power of the 'parish Virgin' and the most recently canonised local saint (Theresa of Lisieux), because they have introduced innovations that make no sense to the locals and because they no longer accept witchcraft as a reality and will not 'unwitch' parishioners. An unbelieving priest: 'sends the bewitched to the psychiatric hospital as if he were a delirious person' (p. 42).

Badone (1989, 1990) shows how baffled, elderly devout Bretons are by the clergy who now work in their parishes, and Bax (1985a, 1985b, 1987, 1988) shows the same in The Netherlands.

It is not only anti-clerical, poorly educated people who mix religion and magic. Patrick Leigh Fermor gives a salutary reminder that a separation between 'religion' and 'magic' is an arbitrary and artificial one.

> I once saw a Cretan priest exorcised by a sorceress of a tiresome sciatica caused by the Evil Eye. For this relief he immediately lit a thanks-giving candle before the ikon of his patron saint.
>
> (Fermor, 1958: 54)

With that Cretan priest in mind, the chapter moves on to magic and popular belief.

MAGIC AND POPULAR BELIEF

There are four themes in this section: popular science ideas, evil eye beliefs, witchcraft beliefs, and folk ideas about vampires, devils and she-devils and other 'spirits'. By 'popular science' or 'ethnoscience', researchers mean ideas held to explain physical, chemical or biological phenomena which are traditional, and do not fit the laboratory science of the school textbook and university lecture. These are studied for a variety of reasons, including their inherent interest (like the 'cheeses' discussed below) and the ways in which adherence to them may impede school science teaching, health education, agricultural advice and other 'modernisations'. If, for example, farmers in a village believe that cows will not eat a particular food, then the bovine nutritionists of the agricultural ministry are unlikely to persuade them to introduce that food into the herds' diet.

Popular or folk science

When Sandra Ott (1979, 1981) was studying French Basque shepherds she discovered that their ethnoscience of conception had
distinguished roots. Ott traces ideas held in Saint-Engrâce of how
conception takes place in the womb, which were that just as rennet is
needed to make milk curdle into cheese, so semen is needed to
curdle in the womb to make a baby. Ott (1979) shows how this idea,
found in the writings of Aristotle, the work of the medieval St
Hildegard (1098–1180) and the belief system of the Occitan village of
Montaillou (Ladurie, 1975), had survived nearly a thousand years.
Favret-Saada (1980) reports a parallel belief about 'cheeses' in the
village where she worked on witchcraft beliefs.

Also in the category of folk science would be the belief of the
Faquir interviewed by Kevin Dwyer (1982: 57) that male circumcision should be done in the morning because: 'the blood isn't
hot. The blood is cold, motionless, and stops flowing right away'.
Not nearly enough research has been done on such ethnoscience,
especially in urban areas (but see Sachs, 1983). Health education
programmes in cities in northern Europe run against folk beliefs
in areas such as AIDS (Aggleton *et al.*, 1988, 1989), and nutrition
(Murcott, 1988). Research on the ethnosciences of Europe is a
major task for the 1990s. Allied to folk beliefs about health and
illness are those surrounding the evil eye.

Evil eye beliefs

Under this heading come a variety of beliefs about envy and the evil
eye, and how they are diagnosed and cured. There is a passionate
debate between Herzfeld (1984) and Galt (1984/5) over whether the
evil eye is 'the same' all around the Mediterranean, which is *not*
rehearsed here. Instead the various fieldwork reports are treated as
reporting roughly equivalent beliefs.

It is difficult to gather data on evil eye beliefs because nobody
wants to appear 'primitive' and 'backward' in the eyes of the
researcher. So Lawrence (1982) found that in the southern
Portuguese town of Vila Branca, younger people were reluctant to
admit that they believed in the evil eye, because to do so would
make them appear 'backward'. However, young children and
babies had protective amulets fixed under their garments, before
a wedding the sign of the cross was painted onto the houses and

garden walls of both bride and groom, and 'curers' still existed to lift the evil eye from its victims. Lawrence did her fieldwork in 1976/77, and the same evil eye beliefs had been reported by Cutileiro (1971). Data such as these suggest beliefs are persistent and relatively stable, although people may be increasingly reluctant to tell middle-class 'city' people about them.

'Envy' is reported as a problem from many cultures. The idea is that if someone is jealous, their envy can cause harm to its object, through gossip (discussed in Chapter 9), witchcraft or sorcery (in the next section), or the evil eye. In some places the 'aggressor', the person who projects the envy or casts the evil eye, is believed to be doing it consciously and deliberately. In others, the 'aggressor' cannot control the force, which attacks victims whether the aggressor wishes to harm them or not. As no-one ever confesses to the researcher that they are an aggressor, researchers only get the stories of *victims*: we know only about what it feels like to be on the receiving end of envy or the evil eye.

Laura, a woman in Vila Cha, believed she suffered from the envy of her neighbours, as did her niece.

> She's miserable here. She's sick with *nervos e barriga* ('nerves' and stomach problems). She's very like me in that the same things upset her in the same way and she has the same health problems . . . It's the atmosphere of *inveja* that's so hard for her here. And for me . . . people are full of *inveja* of me . . . People say things deliberately to upset you, and afterward you become sick with *nervos* and things go 'round and 'round in your head and you have nightmares.
>
> (Cole, 1991: 112)

Envy or the evil eye is invoked not to explain obvious physical injuries or illnesses but to explain recurrent, persistent, vague ill-health that the local doctor cannot 'cure'. Thus Zinovieff (1991a) found that many Nafpliotes had a residual belief in the evil eye (*to mati*) and would blame lethargy or headaches on it. Jealousy or spite will produce an attack of the eye from others.

Stewart (1991) did fieldwork in Apeiranthos on Naxos, in a particularly isolated community of shepherds renowned for their fierceness and hostility to outsiders. Evil eye beliefs still existed there, and it was thought to be 'a projectile form of envy' (p. 232). A hostile stare can strike a person, an animal, or a mechanical device such as a motorbike. Anything which is a valuable family possession, such as children, but also TV sets, is in danger of an attack (p. 232). Symptoms of an attack by the evil eye include feeling persistently tired and lacking in energy, and recurrent headaches. Babies which cry continuously may be thought to have suffered an attack of the evil eye (*to mati*), as are adults who have lost their 'get up and go'.

Because the evil eye is an ever-present danger sensible people protect themselves. Ana in Vila Cha:

> wears a *figa* and a small horn on a chain round her neck, which she says are to protect her from the *inveja*, the evil eye (*mau olhado*) of her neighbours. The *figa* is an amulet in the form of a clenched fist with the thumb placed between the index and middle fingers. She also has a six-pointed star . . . carved on her cement wash tub.
>
> (Cole, 1991: 117)

In the *trulli* country of southern Italy the houses had crosses painted on their roofs to ward off the evil eye (Appel, 1976).

A person who suspects that they are the victim of envy or the evil eye will seek a diagnosis and a cure. In Apeiranthos victims are diagnosed by dropping oil into water – if it coagulates the evil eye has been at work. This diagnosis is reported also from Apulia by Appel (1976). Once a diagnosis has been made, Naxiotes removed the evil eye by saying a prayer (which invoked the Trinity), dropping a cross into a glass of water and then sprinkling the bubbles of water from the cross on oneself. In Portugal, victims may consult a *bruxo* (white witch) who diagnoses the evil eye and cures it (Pina-Cabral, 1986; Cole, 1991). These are discussed in the next section. In some cultures, the evil eye just dissipates, in others it is turned back onto the aggressor.

Evil eye beliefs are found not only among Catholics and Ortho- dox Christians, but also among the Islamic peoples of North Africa and Turkey. Daisy Dwyer (1978: 132–136) describes the evil eye (*L'ain*) beliefs in a traditional Moroccan town (Taroudannt). A newborn baby is protected first with a bundle of spices, minerals and silver (*srira*) tied round its neck or wrist. A careful mother then seeks spiritual protection from a saint, by getting the child's hair cut at the saint's tomb or house of the brotherhood devoted to that saint. The distinctive hairstyle imposed by the saint's cult helps demonstrate the protective care of the saint and ward off the evil eye (and evil spirits or *jnun*). Small children are particularly vulnerable to the evil eye and evil spirits.

More dangerous than the evil eye is witchcraft or sorcery. There are three types of witch or sorcerer around in contemporary Europe: the wicked witch who casts spells on others and causes their misfortunes; the white witch or unwitcher who diagnoses spells and either removes or reverses them; and the pagan: the person who has rejected Christianity for what they believe to be 'older' religions such as Egyptian, Celtic or Norse pantheons or feminist invocations of nature and earth mothers. The latter, studied in the UK by Luhrmann (1989), are intellectually fascinating but beyond the scope of this book. The next section focuses on witches and unwitchers in contemporary Europe.

Witchcraft and sorcery

The oddest, and most maddening book about witchcraft beliefs in contemporary Europe is Favret-Saada (1980). Between 1968 and 1971 Favret-Saada, a sophisticated Paris-based intellectual, did fieldwork in the north-west of France, in an area she protected by calling it only the 'Bocage'. She was faced with a particularly difficult research problem: peasant farmers do not want to discuss beliefs about witchcraft with intellectuals from Paris, because to do so labels them as backward bumpkins, endangers them because witches do not like their victims talking about witchcraft, and renders them liable to be confined to the local psychiatric hospital as deluded, mad, insane.

Gradually Favret-Saada came to realise that unless she believed in witchcraft herself, she would not be able to study it. After collecting some stories of witchcraft she was introduced to Josephine and Jean Babin, who became central figures in her research. Jean was an impotent alcoholic, who had been admitted to the local psychiatric hospital, and whose small farm was suffering because his cows had epizotic abortions and brucellosis. Gradually Favret-Saada discovered that the Babins were convinced that they were being bewitched by a malevolent neighbour, and that they had fixed on Favret-Saada to be their unwitcher. This was marvellous as a way of getting her data, but also very frightening, because in the belief system of the Bocage, the unwitcher is in great danger. He or she takes the magic from the victim and tries to send it boomeranging back onto the witch. If that works, only the evil witch suffers. If the unwitcher is not strong enough, the magic leaves the original victim and attacks the unwitcher instead.

As long as Favret-Saada did not believe in the existence of witch-craft she could 'act' as an unwitcher for the Babins, or pretend to act. However Favret-Saada began to believe that witchcraft was a better explanation of Jean Babin's impotence than anything orthodox psychiatry could offer him, and found herself believing that the witchcraft had indeed been diverted from Jean Babin to her. She began to have accidents as if the witchcraft had indeed been diverted from the Babins to herself. This was the anthropologist 'going native' with a vengeance.

Essentially, Favret-Saada argues that witchcraft beliefs and the ways in which Bocage families tried to divert witchcraft from victims 'worked' better as therapy and as resolution for family problems than psychiatry did. Her 1989 article is a much clearer exposition of her ideas, that the tensions generated inside families are diffused onto unspecified neighbours by the unwitcher. This is a typical anthropological interpretation of witchcraft beliefs: they are a way of highlighting tensions in the social structure.

Equivalent to the unwitcher in the Bocage is the Portuguese *bruxo*, who diagnoses and cures the evil eye. Cole (1991) and Pina-Cabral (1986) both offer accounts of how victims of *inveja* consult *bruxos* – or rather *bruxas* because many of them are wise women. Pina-Cabral says that 'white witches remain central figures in peasant life' (p. 189). There are now two kinds of white witches. There is the traditional one with a 'local clientele usually con-sisting of poor, rural people' (p. 191) and a new kind, who has appeared and taken over much of the work since the 1960s, and is 'urban, bourgeois, often educated, and bases his or her work on many different kinds of information' (p. 191).

The rise of the new urban white witches is due to post-Vatican II priests withdrawing exorcism from their parishioners. The new white witches live in cities – because they are symbolising their modern, urban status – and benefit from being in an anonymous town. Clients prefer to come in from a gossipy village in anonymity, and rely on taxi-drivers to recommend a *bruxo/a*. Pina-Cabral (1986: 192–193) tells the story of a woman going to a *bruxa* to discover if her husband was going to pass his driving test and being impressed when she was told he would, but would have to emigrate to Brazil. A couple in Paco went to a *bruxa* in Oporto because their shop was not prospering. It had been attacked by *feitico* (sorcery). The *bruxa* came to the shop, divined where the *feiticio* was hidden, and told them to cast it into the sea ('it' was, to Pina-Cabral's eyes, 'nondescript' dust) (p. 195). Pina-Cabral sees the growth of new urban *bruxos/as* as both replacing the priest and providing a day out, in addition to their functions in dealing with peoples' problems.

The final set of supernatural phenomena to be considered are vampires, devils, she-devils, and other spirits.

Vampires, devils and spirits

Many supernatural beings swarm over Europe. Pina-Cabral (1987) has described the enchanted mooresses who haunt northern Portugal, Holmes (1989: 154–163) found the good witches (*benedans* or *stregoni buoni*) still went out at night to fight off evil spirits in northern Italy. Du Boulay (1982) tells how an improperly buried body can turn into a vampire, and Stewart (1991) is packed with material on vampires and other *exotika* on Naxos. Devils and she-devils may possess the unwary, like the woman crawling to the church on Tinos (Dubisch, 1990). Crapanzano (1980) is an account of Tuhami's possession by the she-devil A'isha Qandisha, who appears as a beautiful woman and captures men unless they spot that she has camel's feet under her dress and escape her clutches. Many of these 'creatures' survive in stories, which are told as entertainment and as a form of social control (for example, to keep people at home after dark).

These are certainly entertaining, and modern equivalents keep developing, studied by folklorists as 'urban legends'. Delamont (1989, 1991) gives examples of such legends told by British teenagers. The belief in the existence of covens of satanists in Britain ritually abusing children, held strongly by some educated professionals (Victor, 1993), shows that no sophisticated city-dweller should disparage the Portuguese villager who 'saw' an enchanted mooress.

Beliefs in both religious and magical phenomena are commonplace in Europe, and have economic, social and practical consequences.

SUGGESTED READING/ACTIVITY

Charles Stewart's (1991) *Demons and the Devil*, and S. Delamont's (1991) 'The HIT LIST and other horror stories', give two perspectives on popular belief systems.

Chapter 9

The gossips of the town
Sex and gender in contemporary Europe

... I pass and thou art gone,
So fast in fire the great boat beats the seas.
But slowly fade, soft Island! Ah to know
Thy town and who the gossips of thy town.

(Flecker, 1947: 106)

INTRODUCTION

In Flecker's poem on the island of Hyali, the sex of the town gossips is not made explicit: it is however, a cherished sexual stereotype that women gossip. This chapter examines such stereotypes of masculinity and femininity.

It is very difficult for the likely readers of this book to *understand* the material in this chapter, and to suspend their judgements and maintain cultural relativity. The whole issue of relations between the sexes is personal and emotional, and very hard to think about objectively. Equally, these issues are hard for anthropologists to research properly, and often difficult for informants to talk about. Then the whole area is complicated by the ways in which informants may tell the researcher what *ought* to happen, or what they *wish* did happen, rather than what actually goes on. Men and women may have different understandings of how their society works, and where the power lies.

There are eight themes in this chapter. It opens with an explanation of 'muted groups', a useful explanatory framework for understanding sex roles. Then there is a section on how we can conceptualise sex segregation and sex equality. Gossip is the focus of the third section, followed by a note on how the sex of the anthropologist relates to the data he or she can collect. The main body of the chapter is a description of some extremely sex-segregated societies, the honour–shame system found in southern Europe and beliefs about proper male and female behaviour. Finally, the paradox of femininity and sex equality is examined.

MUTED GROUPS

The idea of muted groups is particularly helpful for grasping material on gender in Europe. The idea comes from the work of Shirley Ardener and her late husband Edwin Ardener, an anthropologist who had done his own research in Africa but was also interested in Europe having supervised McDonald (1989) and Chapman (1978). These ideas of dominant and muted groups were put forward in Ardener (1972) and further developed in Ardener (1975). They have subsequently inspired a set of volumes emanating from a series of women's studies seminars in Oxford, published as Shirley Ardener (1975, 1978, 1981), Burman (1979), Jacobus (1979), Hutter and Williams (1981), Holden (1983), Callan and Ardener (1984), and Hirschon (1984). Shirley Ardener (1985) has written a brief reflection on the decade of publications from this group. Delamont and Duffin (1978: 11–14) illuminated material on nineteenth-century feminist campaigns, and Delamont (1989) focused on teenage girls and their world view, via muted group theory.

Edwin and Shirley Ardener had studied a tribe in the Cameroons where the men and women lived very separate lives. The Ardeners came to the conclusion that too many anthropologists had focused on the dominant male model of how a society worked, and ignored the possibility that other groups in the culture (such as subordinate men, women, religious minorities, ethnic minorities, or outcasts) might have a different understanding of the ways in which their culture operated. So the pictures of societies brought home by anthropologists were too often the dominant male model to the neglect of other models that existed in that culture. The Ardeners coined the term 'muted group' to cover those sub-sections of any culture whose model of how their society worked was 'drowned out', 'swamped' by the dominant group. They argued that there were at least three good reasons for studying the world views of muted groups. First, the behaviour of a muted group may be determined by *their* world view, not that of the dominant group. (This is, for example, the case with gypsies in modern Europe.) Second, the world view of a muted group may be important for throwing the dominant group's model into relief, as it is often necessary to see what an opposition believes in order to grasp what the group in power adhere to. Third, the ideas of the muted group may be fascinating in their own right. When women are the muted group, all three reasons can apply simultaneously.

Shirley Ardener (1975) has expressed the ideas of dominant and muted groups in the following way. It is argued that every group in a society generates and shares common models of society and of sections of society,

> a society may be dominated or overdetermined by the model (or models) generated by one dominant group within the system. This dominant model may impede the free expression of alternative models of their world which subdominant groups may possess, and perhaps may even inhibit the very generation of such models. Groups dominated in this sense find it necessary to structure their world through the model (or models) of the dominant group, transforming their own models as best they can in terms of the received ones.

The Ardeners have suggested that women typically form such a muted, inarticulate group. Thus, models are said to exist at different levels of consciousness and generality. The Ardeners suggest that while both dominant and muted groups probably generate ideas of social reality at deep levels, the ideas of the dominant group so blanket the surface of everyday life that the muted group is likely to find its generation of surface ideas inhibited by the blanket coverage. It is not clear quite how muted groups adjust to the dislocation between their deep models and the surface models of the dominant group, but it is argued that they will learn to express their own deepest ideas in terms of the dominant group's surface ideas. Thus a muted group transforms 'their own unconscious perceptions into such conscious ideas as will accord with those generated by the dominant group'. Such transformations may require the investment of 'a great deal of disciplined mental energy'. This expenditure of energy may well explain the conservative nature of many muted groups' world views: their attachment to models which leave them at a disadvantage. For, as Shirley Ardener argues, it is not surprising if people cling to a dearly-won accommodation and fear the prospect of a fresh start.

Ardener argues that studies of the position of women frequently illustrate how women are placed in an inferior category in the predominant system of a given society compared to the men of the society. However, even after the relative position of women in the structure has been documented and established, there is another fruitful area for research. This is the whole topic of the unclear, vague and probably repressed alternative theories which women have about the world and, perhaps even more interestingly, about themselves. It is these, and the relationships between them and the dominant ideologies, which form the topics for this chapter.

There is also a question that can legitimately be asked once a researcher has discovered that the dominant group's model of their society is not the only one that exists in it. If there is a muted group with a different model, the researcher can find out whether the dominant group recognises that the muted group *have* an alternative world view, and if so how they regard it. (For example, is it seen as wrong, perverted, mistaken, ignorant, malicious or what?) The muted group normally have a good grasp of the dominant model, because they have to understand it in order to survive, but the reverse is often not the case.

A good example of dominant and muted group models of a society can be found in Berkowitz's (1984) analysis of the family in southern Italy. She argues that the dominant model, held by men and in public by women too, is that men are the bosses of their homes and families. However, the women actually are the *real* power in the household, and merely pretend that the man is to keep the peace, make him feel good, and maintain the illusion of a patriarchal society. As one informant told Cronin (1970: 76): 'the husband is like the government of Rome, all pomp; the wife is like the mafia, all power'. This is a Sicilian proverb, quoted with approval by Berkowitz (1984). When studying the beliefs and practices surrounding men, masculinity, women and feminity, it is vital to separate the views of the dominant group from those of the muted group(s). It is also important to distinguish between sex segregation and sex equality.

SEX SEGREGATION AND SEX EQUALITY

Many of the cultures studied by anthropologists practice strict sex segregation: typically women have a sphere of home, church and shopping, while men are expected to be outside in the fields or at work, and then with other men in a bar, inn, café or pub, or in the public spaces such as the square, waterfront or street corner. It is very easy to equate such segregated sex roles with inequality between men and women, but life is not that simple. A society can have rigidly segregated sex roles, but both men and women can believe they are equal in it. Another society could have men and women mixing freely, but be riddled with inequalities.

Equality and segregation are two quite distinct dimensions. As Figure 9.1 shows, there are four possible ways for the sexes to be ordered in any culture, because they can be highly segregated or hardly segregated at all, while at the same time highly unequal or relatively equal in terms of power, autonomy, wealth, and so on. In this model Quadrant A represents a society in which the sexes are segregated and are unequal, such as rural Sicily, the Sarakatsani or the gypsy world. Quadrant B represents a culture where the sexes are rarely together, but there is not a clear hierarchy of power, such as the traditional farming system of the Basque country as described in Douglass (1975). Quadrant C is a culture where the sexes mingle but one is dominant over the other, and Quadrant D one where the sexes mingle *and* are equal. In modern Britain, there is a widespread but simplistic belief that the more segregated the sex roles are the more 'oppressed' women are, and that the road to sex equality is for men and women to do the same tasks alongside each other. That is, if we want sex equality in Britain we should move towards Quadrant D. Thus in Britain we have allowed Wrens to go to sea, and policewomen to pound the beat and ride in the patrol cars alongside men. So the élite men-only London club is seen as an anachronism, as old-fashioned, and women who want access to them believe this would be a form of advancement towards equality. In this belief system, single-sex schools, hospitals or leisure pursuits are 'old-fashioned'. (Separatist, radical feminists are unusual in rejecting this model of sex equality.) There is a widespread belief in contemporary Britain that in the private sphere a married couple ought to want to spend time together, talking and sharing things, including the birth of babies, the DIY and the housework. Sharing everything is actually a very new idea, and is not universal across social classes in the UK. There are upper-class and working-class marriages in which the partners do not believe in such 'sharing', but in the other model, of segregated sex roles. Bott (1971) found that many working-class couples

Segregation
High

Inequality
High   A   B   Low
                                  C   D

                                 Low

Figure 9.1 Sex segregation and sex equality

functioned perfectly well with segregated sex roles, and as long as both sexes are happy with that model, it is not a bar to sex equality in itself.

Equality may not come from the sexes being integrated or inequality from segregating them. It may be hard to accept that large areas of Europe have no ideal of companionate marriage, and instead believe in rigid segregation of the sexes. For the purposes of this chapter, please suspend any ideas you have about women's equality or 'modernity', and concentrate on understanding the belief systems anthropologists have discovered. Remember that Switzerland, a 'modern' country, only gave women the vote in 1971. On Tory Island, off the coast of Ireland it is common for married couples to live apart, each staying on in their childhood home. Of fifty-one married couples in 1963, ten were still in their natal homes. This was seen as entirely sensible, because the two families were not disturbed by a 'child' leaving or a spouse moving in. Fox (1978) obviously found this odd – he had the idea that getting married involves living in the same house – but the Tory Islanders did not, and it was their island and their lives.

GOSSIP

Gossip is one way in which male and female roles are enforced and reinforced. In Ballybran (Scheper-Hughes, 1979) married couples were not seen together in public. When one young couple broke these rules – for example by sitting together in church; the husband was attacked.

Word spread that he was putting on city airs and 'acting queer'. After the birth of a child when Dennis took to promenading on the strand with the baby buggy, criticism turned to vicious ridicule.

(p. 108)

Dennis gave up trying to be a companionate husband and soon he and his wife were no longer seen together.

Gossip controls – or rather fear of gossip controls – many things other than male and female behaviour, but it is particularly aroused by real or imagined deviations from ideal masculinity or femininity, or lapses from that society's standards of respectability, fidelity and modesty. Parman (1990: 102) reports the controlling functions of gossip in Gaell in the Outer Hebrides:

It is difficult for people raised in the anonymity of an urban environment to imagine living in a setting in which you are continually confronted with the living memory . . . of your mistakes and failures.

As Parman points out: 'the watchful neighbour, the gossiping tongue . . . is an important element in social control. Even the thought that someone might think you were doing something keeps behaviour circumspect' (pp. 102–103). The vital thing is to protect the *appearance* of your self, your family, your household. As an elderly bachelor, with whom gossip linked Parman herself, put it: 'if you maintain the proper image, you can do anything you want' (p. 103). Parman had been romantically linked to this bachelor because she once spent the night at his house not alone, but in a party, in a society where all night visiting was 'a common form of socializing', but her 'presence was advertised' (p. 103). Gossip spread and: 'My family was scandalized . . . because they were afraid of how the gossip about me might reflect upon them' (p. 103). Her 'family' means, not her American kin, but the locals she was living with whose reputation could be damaged by her behaviour even though she was 'only' the lodger.

These are Celtic examples, but du Boulay (1974) reports similar pressures in Ambeli, where there is a 'continual battle between secrecy and curiosity that is waged between the various families' (p. 202). So everyone is trying to protect their own privacy and secrecy, while finding out about other people. Both sexes gossip, although it is believed that women 'do nothing but gossip' (p. 205). Du Boulay points out that there is nothing else to do in Ambeli:

no cinema, no chance of dressing up and 'going out', no concerts, books, theatres or television – in fact no form of prepared entertainment at all, except for a radio which not all houses possess.

(1974: 205)

Zinovieff (1991a) did fieldwork in Nafplion, Greece, in 1985–87. She has analysed how gossip functions to define who is a Nafpliote (outsiders are not privy to gossip about Nafplion, nor are they the subject of gossip) and to control behaviour – especially women's behaviour. Initially she did not experience Nafplion as a gossip-ridden place but: 'later, I too felt the claustrophobia that the existence of gossip can produce. It seems as though *nothing* one does may remain secret' (p. 121). Women feared gossip about 'alleged sexual misdemeanours', while men dreaded gossip about them 'lacking the strength and control which a man should have' (p. 122).

Similarly, Loizos (1981: 29) points out that neither sex can ever relax, because:

as vigilant, thoughtful family members, they were ever on the look-out for those tiny scraps of information which might serve towards the advancement of their own family, or what was very nearly the same thing, towards the decline of another house.

Gossip is, then, part of upholding your family's honour and therefore denigrating other peoples'. Bailey (1971a) is a collection of papers on village life in Spain, Italy, Austria and France where gossip is a major form of social control. As Bailey introduces the theme of the volume he uses data from the fieldwork of Susan Hutson (1971): 'Housewives in Valloire avoid being seen talking to one another' (Bailey, 1971b: 1). This is because if women are seen talking to one another, everyone assumes they are 'indulging in *mauvaise langue* – gossip, malice, "character assassination"' (p. 1). Men seen talking are assumed to be engaged in *bavarder*: 'a friendly, sociable, light-hearted, good natured, altruistic exchange of news' (p. 1).

Women therefore try not to be seen talking to other women. Blaxter (1971) reports the same belief from Auguste in the French Pyrenees, and Heppenstall (1971) an equivalent distinction between *plaudern* (good-natured chatter) and *tratschen* (gossip) from Sankt Martin in Austria. In fact, both sexes 'gossip', but men and women share the fiction that only women do so. So not only does gossip act as a form of control over men and women but beliefs about what men and women do are embodied as beliefs about gossip. Many aspects of sex and gender are equally circular, as the rest of the chapter shows. The next theme is the inter-relation of the sex of the anthropologist and the data on sex roles that he or she can collect.

SEX ROLES AND FIELDWORK

The more strictly segregated the sex roles in a culture, the more difficult it is for a male anthropologist to study women's lives, and discover how they understand their world. As Susan Rogers (1975: 126) points out, much of the anthropology of Europe has been biased towards accounts of men's lives.

> The fieldwork method itself is partly to blame for this. Because most societies are strictly sex-segregated, and most anthropo-logists are men, access to information about women has largely been limited to what male informants know or are willing to tell.

Women are able to collect some data on men, but not vice versa: 'Women anthropologists, unlike their male colleagues, have an ambiguous social gender in many field situations, allowing them access to social domains and informants of either or both sexes' (Rogers, 1975: 126).

Loizos's (1981) account of his first fieldwork visit to a Cypriot village reveals how hard it was for a single man from London to understand sex segregation, and harder to find out about women's lives. Giovannini (1986) is an account of a woman researcher's diffi-culties in doing fieldwork on men in a segregated Sicilian village.

The Sarakatsani are probably the most extreme case of a division of labour by sex in a Christian people in Europe. Campbell (1964) lived with the Sarakatsani in 1954, with his wife Sheila.

> My wife did share the fieldwork with me and given the regime of extreme modesty on which the reputation of unmarried girls depended, as well as the prudent behaviour of married women, it is doubtful if I could have talked freely on matters which concerned women if my wife had not been there.
>
> (Campbell, 1992: 153)

Brandes (1992) settled in Monteros in 1975 with his wife and two daughters. He too was able to learn from them about women's lives, as well as men's from his own interaction with men. As he stresses male researchers in a segregated community like Monteros cannot spend time with women.

> For a man to spend conspicuous hours of conversation in public with an unrelated woman is to challenge her husband's, father's or brother's legitimate protective role, and to place her honour in question.
>
> (p. 33)

Just as Scheper-Hughes (1979) could not drink in the Ballybran pub, Brandes could not talk to the grandmother who sold the family chickens without damaging the social fabric. It is against this background that the research on sex and gender has to be understood.

SEX ROLES: SEGREGATED AND INTEGRATED

This section illustrates the wide range of different sex-role systems across western Europe, starting with three fiercely segregated and unequal ones: the Sarakatsani of northern Greece in the 1950s, the Maniot Greeks in the 1920s and the Spanish gypsies in the 1960s.

The Sarakatsani had, in the 1950s, one of the most rigid sex role systems found in Europe, with women apparently subordinated and segregated. Campbell's (1964) account reads like a stereotype of women's lives in an Islamic country. The role of women is essentially private, domestic and chaste before marriage, private, domestic and faithful after it. If before her marriage a women violates these norms, the honour of her whole family, her father and brothers, is stained; if after, her husband and *his* family are ruined by her lapse.

Sarakatsani women could be seen as both segregated (they did *not* share tasks with men, but spent their time with other women doing women's work) and subordinated. In theory at least, before marriage a woman was under the control of her father and brothers, who could kill her if she was 'immodest', and on marriage passed to the control of her husband, his father and brothers, and his mother, who controlled the work she had to do. Reading about the life of a Sarakatsani woman in the 1950s produces a clear sense of both segregation and submission.

Similar draconian standards governed sex roles in other parts of Greece before the Second World War. Seremetakis (1991:

144–148), in her study of the Mani, recounts the story, from the 1920s, of how the male relatives of a beautiful heiress, Vengelio, killed her when she became pregnant outside marriage. Her parents had taken her to the regional capital and hidden her, but her male kin held a lottery, and the young cousin who drew the short straw killed her with a shotgun. Maniot women were kept as segregated and subordinate as Sarakatsani in the pre-war years. Many fieldworkers have been told such stories, especially by older people who may tell researchers these tales of a 'golden age' when morals were strict and families controlled their members tightly as part of a general rhetorical strategy: to make the past of their village sound splendid and ultra-respectable. Herzfeld (1983) argues this for highland Crete, and it may also be true of the Mani. However, even if we allow for rhetorical exaggeration in such stories, the ideal sex-role system is clear: segregation and male domination.

Like the Sarakatsani, the gypsies (*gitanos/gitanas*) studied by Quintana and Floyd (1972) in Andalusia and by Mulcahy (1976) in northern Spain had one of the strongest divisions of labour by sex reported from a Christian community. Men, who worked as unskilled building labourers, and women, who *never* worked for non-gypsies for wages, but scavenged discarded consumer goods from middle-class and industrial neighbourhoods, dressed in ways that emphasised their contrasting roles. Men who have to go outside the gypsy world among those who are not of the gypsy race (*la raza gitana*) and work among *payos* obey their rules and dress neutrally to do so. Women, who go into the *payo* world to scavenge always go in gypsy clothes and with their children. Among themselves young *gitano* men dress *machismo* which means hair in long flamenco style, tight trousers, pointed shoes, studded belts, wristbands, fringed cowboy shirts worn open to expose the chest. Men also carry a *baston* (cane). This macho style is toned down by older men. Males all smoke coarse black tobacco, engage in ritualised beer/wine drinking, and guitar playing in an aggressive style. Little boys mimic this behaviour. Gypsy women dressed in a very unprovocative way, deliberately dowdy. The female uniform is skirts and jumpers, with hair pulled back into a knot, and an apron all the time. The only deviation from dowdiness is gold jewellery, such as large earrings and medals on chains, a display of wealth which can be pawned when times are hard. Women gypsies dressed in a deliberately unsexy way, with the apron symbolising domesticity.

Men and women spend little time together; each sex spends time with same-sex peers. Men expect to police the behaviour of their wives, daughters and sisters, with violence if 'necessary'. A woman who is thought to be sexually immoral will not be able to stay among gypsies; she is killed or driven away.

These segregated and tightly controlled sex roles among Spanish gypsies are exactly the opposite of non-*gitano* stereotypes. *Payo* society believes that gypsies are sexually promiscuous, and gypsy women are symbols of 'free' women, especially since the opera *Carmen*. In fact gypsies have very strict standards of female chastity – so that gypsy girls are married very young, at 12 or 13, while their families can ensure they are still virgins – and married gypsy women go around in groups with children to chaperone them.

The Sarakatsani, gypsies and the Mani of the 1920s are the most extreme end of a continuum of sex role behaviours In farming and fishing communities the labour of both sexes is needed to keep the family going (which is why peasant farmers need wives) and women are valued if they are hardworking and thrifty, but still have to behave modestly enough to avoid any gossip. This is usually summarised by anthropologists of the Mediterranean area as the 'honour and shame system': a belief system in which the honour or respectability of a family is dependent on the man behaving like a man and, even more important, 'his' women showing modesty, chastity and fidelity.

For example, when Simon (1976) was studying an isolated mountain village in rural Corsica, he found the traditional value system of *onore* v. *vergogna* still in place. Men told him: '*Fatti onore chi vergogna un ti ne manca*' which translated poetically means 'Honour shames those who lack it'. This is a classic statement of a belief system found in southern Portugal, southern Spain, southern Italy and the islands of Malta, Cyprus, Corsica and Sicily.

Cucchiari (1988: 429) points out that women are kept in a double bind by the 'patriarchal order' of Sicilian society.

> On the one hand, marriage is one of the few honourable ways to a measure of autonomy and respectability for women, but, on the other, courtship is a risky game for women because they have little control over the rules or outcome. In short, courtship and marriage are institutions that dramatically confront young Sicilian women with their vulnerability, dependence and power-lessness. Collapsed engagements, for example, can all too easily doom a woman to spinsterhood.

When Cutileiro (1971) wrote *A Portuguese Rural Society*, his study of a village in the south, a particularly risky period for a young woman's reputation (and hence that of her family) was courtship. A young woman needs to find a husband while keeping her spotless reputation. Cutileiro collected the story of one stormy courtship (*namoro*). At this period in this village once a girl was engaged she was stuck with that fiancé. If the engagement was broken off her honour was irretrievably damaged, so she had to be modest and faithful, and hang on at all costs. He tells the story of Penelope who had been engaged for five years to a man working away from the village (including two years in the navy on national service). After his two years in the navy he wrote and broke the engagement. Later he was heard to be in Lisbon getting engaged to a girl there. His family intervened and brought him home because Penelope had been totally moral and faithful and they did not want their status or hers damaged. He then married her because she 'knew how to wait for me', and had proved herself a 'good girl'. There had been *no* gossip about her, so she must have spent five very dull years, always chaperoned, and mostly at her home, sewing the linen for her bottom drawer.

The 'honour and shame' value system is usually found with a strong division of labour and segregated use of space in the village, town or city. Lison-Tolosana's (1966) study of Belmont de los Caballeros, a village in Aragon, has the common phenomenon: women have total control inside the household, but are confined to it apart from shopping and church-going. Men have public spaces, coffee houses and the village square, and control over the behaviour of their families when in public. So if a young man or woman is seen behaving improperly it reflects on their father's lack of proper responsibility. Similar patterns are reported from Escalona in Andalusia (Uhl, 1985), where the local proverb ran: *La mujer es para la casa y el hombre es para el campo* (Women are meant for the house and men are meant for the fields) (p. 130).

Uhl argues that in the 1980s, among the under-25s segregations were seen as an old-fashioned pattern, and the 35–40-year-olds told her that they had seen the pattern begin to break down when women began to go into bars, with their fiancés or even with women friends. Bars *had* been a rigidly 'male' territory, especially in Andalusia. Other researchers also studying southern Europe in the 1980s do not seem so confident that the segregations are breaking down, or that bars are losing their central place in male culture. Driessen (1983: 125) says: 'the bar or café is a focal institution of public life, the stage *par excellence* of male sociability'. In the town he studied the ideal male: 'is tough (*duro*), strong (*fuerte*), formal (*sobrio*), autonomous and undisputed head of the household. He supports his family, guards the family honour, and is seldom at home' (p. 125).

The bar is the place where these characteristics are displayed in a ritualised way. There were nine bars in the small town, including one for the local élite (called by the workers the 'fat club') and five traditional bars. In the traditional bars the majority of the men display their masculinity to each other by standing rounds of drinks, by telling stories, and *cachondeo* a competitive form of joking. Actual violence is not valued, but the potential for aggression held in by the man's self-control is highly regarded. Driessen (1983: 131) suggests that these rituals of male sociability in bars are particularly popular with day-labourers and the rest of the working class, because:

> Rituals of masculinity in cafés act to mask the reality of the day-labourer's dependence on the female members of his household and his weak economic and political position in local society.

Some scholars went so far as to call the honour–shame system, *the* unifying feature of Mediterranean Europe (Pitt-Rivers, 1977; Gilmore and Gwynne, 1985; Gilmore, 1987a and 1987b). Before discussing whether the system *is* a unifying factor along the north coast of the Mediterranean, it is important to recognise that where the honour–shame system did exist, it was not simply a way of oppressing women. By the standards of an undergraduate at a British university, the life of Penelope in Vila Velha appears restricted and oppressed. However, such a system also places strains on men, for they too are required to behave only in one way: macho and vigilant. Honour is also important for men, who must not *only* protect the reputation and chastity of 'their' women, but also provide for them (feed and clothe and *dower* dependent daughters).

The pressures on the majority of working-class men, especially the day-labourers, as summarised by Driessen (1983) from the agrotown he studied, and his analysis of their use of the all-male bar culture as a way of handling those pressures, is very similar to that of Press (1979: 86–90) in his account of male bars in Seville, which are a man's refuge and: 'business office, labour exchange, and social club' (p. 187). In the *barrio* Press studied there were 110 bars in an area eight city blocks square. Each bar has its regulars (men) who are there several times a day, sometimes for several hours. There: 'the Sevillano can drink on credit, tell dirty jokes, share gossip and ogle the girls who pass'. The man can also buy condoms from a salesman (less embarrassing than from a woman in a shop) and lottery tickets. The bar owner will take telephone messages, and for the self-employed, offers of work are made. Upper-class men have bars too, but they have nicer housing, and spend more time at home, or at friends' homes, than the poor men do.

Brandes (1980, 1981, 1985, 1987, 1992) has devoted a good number of his publications on the Castilian and the Andalusian communities he has studied to sex roles, and especially to the (working-class) men's folklore and 'ethnoscience' about women. The men in Monteros, the Andalusian agrotown, held very strongly stereotyped views about women, compounded of fear, loathing and longing.

The honour of men who have few skills and little job security or wealth is precarious, and is partly maintained by adherence to stereotypes about 'inferior' beings such as women (and gypsies). Brandes's (1980) and Driessen's (1983) analyses are supported by Marvin's (1986, 1988) work on Andalusian cockfights and bullfights, both arenas in which masculine bravery is displayed, and Murphy (1983a, 1983b) who deals with how teenage boys pass into manhood, and therefore establish their masculinity. In the Seville Barrio Macareno, there were three 'styles' of adolescent masculinity: *santito, golfo, tio*. The *santito* (the little saint) is a mother's boy, a weed and a wet. He is pale because he stays indoors and atttends church with his mother, dresses in clothes adults have chosen for him and he has no 'balls'. A *golfo* is a teenage boy beyond the control of his family (Murphy translates it as 'scoundrel'). He dresses in the extremes of teenage fashion, and is always out on the streets, never at home. The *tio* (a 'regular guy' in Murphy's terms) manages the balancing act: he is on the streets enough to show he has separated from his mother, but is not running wild to the despair of his family.

Much of the literature on the honour and shame system has been based on Spain, especially Andalusia. However, there is evidence from other southern European societies that similar beliefs are held. Men and women should be kept apart, in order to remain uncontaminated by each other. Attempts to integrate men and women are viewed with suspicion. The strength of feeling can

be gauged from a Maltese primary teacher interviewed by
Darmanin (1990). Miss Ximenes had taught in a girls' primary
school, amalgamated into a mixed one. Both staffroom and play-
ground relationships became problematic for Miss Ximenes.
Darmanin writes:

> The amalgamation of the single sex girls' primary school with the
> boys' primary can be seen as a critical incident for Miss Ximenes.
> The second day of term, a chance playground remark about the
> teachers getting on well together was followed by a more detailed
> account when I showed interest in the initial remark. Miss
> Ximenes said that when the schools were single sex, she and the
> other women teachers used to 'have a great time'. Staffroom
> humour was more unguarded and even the ex-headmistress would
> join in. On occasion, the neighbouring male teachers from the
> boys' school were asked to join the female staff. A fictitious engage-
> ment, followed by a wedding, was held between Mr Adami (now of
> Minsija, Year 6G) and the ex-headteacher (now Head of Primary
> A). Miss Ximenes gets on with the male teachers, but 'it was more
> fun when it was women only'.

This is quite typical of how, when the sexes are kept separate,
certain joking relationships and 'symbolic' ties between men and
women can be encouraged and enjoyed. Uhl (1985) describes a
(lapsed) system of ritualised special friendships in Andalusia.
Once there is official mixing, such joking relationships may wither.
Darmanin (1990) goes on:

> Miss Ximenes found pupil–pupil relationships in the newly
> mixed schools raised difficulties for her too. Her critique of the
> amalgamation extends to the effects it has on the children. Her
> explicit objection to mixed schooling is precipitated by
> Godwin's whispered remark to Maryanne on the 13th October,
> and following a heavy storm in which a roof collapsed on a
> married couple and killed them as they were in bed. Godwin
> tells Maryanne, who then tells the teacher 'I wish the roof would
> fall on us as we are in bed, and you would be in your knickers'.
> Miss Ximenes is worried about the moral tone of her pupils and
> spends the lesson in a sermon in which she describes the moral
> code she expects them to follow. In keeping with her custodial
> orientation to the children and her specific religious beliefs, she
> concludes the session with prayers and the aside to me:

In break, I'm not going to let them play together. God knows what they'll do. At home they can do what they like, but not here, during the break. Me, that's why I'm against it, mixed schooling at this age. We're not English, we're Latins and it's different.

This comment, 'we're Latins and it's different', is similar to the explanation offered when Loizos (1981: 30) was told by an uncle in Argaki: 'We hope we are Europeans in most things . . . but in matters of honour – that is, where our women are concerned – we are happy to be Middle-Easterners.' Loizos initially found the sex segregation very strange:

It was easy enough to remark the absence of women from 'public life' – the coffee shops and the square . . . the deeper meaning of that absence came through to me only slowly, like the ghostly image of the photographic print appearing in the developing bath.

(1981: 28)

Gradually Loizos began to understand these rules.

Mealtimes afforded other clues. In most houses the women never spoke to me at meals before I spoke to them, and did not sit to eat with the men . . . After meals, men at leisure did not sit and talk to their wives. They left smartly for the coffee shops.

(1981: 28)

Women were expected to be in the house, men to be in the fields, or in one of the towns, or in their village coffee house. Loizos heard about an honourable man in Argaki, the father of Stasa, who was married to Loizos's cousin Pakis. Stasa's father had seven daughters and one young son. This meant there was only one man to protect the respectability of eight women. Although in all contexts he was a 'calm and reasonable' (p. 30) man, whenever he heard of any challenge to his daughters' (and hence *his*) respectability he reacted violently. One day a boy at Stasa's school 'told her he quite liked her' (p. 30) so her father beat the boy to show she had a respectable family. Another time Stasa and a sister were taken to the beach by their father 'like the city girls' (p. 29), and put on swimsuits. A boy commented to Stasa 'O, you are very beautiful' so her father 'got angry and hit him with a bottle' (p. 29).

As in Cyprus, so too in Greece. In the farming villages there are pressures on a man to be responsible and fulfil his duties. The virginity of daughters is a symbolic matter, as Machin (1983: 108) explains for rural Crete: 'Virginity is highly regarded as a symbol of the honour of the family.' An honourable man accepts his obligations. In the mountains of Crete, Herzfeld's (1985) men got honour (p. 124) by knowing how to wield a knife, to dance well, being good at exchanging ritual verse insults, by being able to eat meat conspicuously whenever possible, by keeping his word, but also profiting from bargains. A real man must stand up to insults, protect his family from threats, keep the family at a proper economic standard, dispense hospitality, deprecate that hospitality, and show clever humour. In Apeiranthos, an isolated village on Naxos, men who are shepherds should be 'indefatigable and clever, able to cover great distances on foot, cunning is another very strong requirement, and to be full of guile' (Stewart, 1991: 62–63). Popular stories celebrated prowess at sheep stealing – less for gain than for the daring and skill of the theft. Ernestine Friedl's (1962) Greek village – Vasilika – has a verb, *kamarono* – which means giving your daughter an adequate dowry, and men can feel honourable in old age if they have set up all their daughters properly.

So in the cultures where the honour–shame system operates a man gets status by being out of his home with other men, and displaying the behaviours that are of value in men to other men. The ideal is that a man controls 'his' women, if necessary by violence, but it is also the case that the woman is in control of the home, and she can ruin the reputation of her husband (but only at the cost of her own). If in southern Europe there was strict sex segregation, theoretical male superiority with an emphasis on the *ideal* of the wife who does not do field work or take paid employment, and a strong emphasis on honour and shame, northern Europe also had the sex segregation, but more often had economic systems in which the outdoor labour of both sexes was expected and necessary, and lacked the obsessive concern with virginity and adultery reported from southern Europe. Northern Portugal certainly does not have, and has not had for a century, the honour–shame system found in southern Europe. Thus O'Neill (1987) and Brettell (1985) both report high levels of illegitimacy, with poorer women living in villages with illegitimate children lacking public respect but certainly not ostracised. However, this does not mean that men and women mix freely before marriage, or spend time together after it, or that there is 'sex equality', although there may well be a strong value placed on women's labour, which is why the 'bride famine' is such a disaster in the Basque country, Brittany and rural Ireland.

Most anthropologists report from northern Europe that there, too, men have ways of demonstrating their prowess as men, but male prowess, masculine success, *machismo* may be demonstrated in different ways in different cultures. Ott (1981) found that the French Basque shepherds she studied in 1976/77 had relatively equal sex roles, with men up in the hills throughout the summer with the sheep while the women kept the household going in the settlement. Ott worked among the men in the hills with the flocks of sheep, where a man's status is dependent on how well he looks after the sheep and his mountain cheese. In the mountains, men milk the sheep, and that is where men make cheese. In Sainte Engrâce the male role in cheese making is analogous to women's role in making babies. A man's prowess is visible from the mountain cheeses he makes which are displayed proudly, to be judged by other men. A man too old to go into the hills loses status, and is believed to lose all his sexual potency, and his ability to father children, when he no longer has the power to make mountain cheese (Ott, 1981: 205–208).

Most of the traditional farming and fishing communities of northern Europe had a strong tradition of sex segregation reported by Scheper-Hughes (1979) for rural Ireland, McDonald (1989) for Brittany, for Germany (Golde, 1975) and for Alpine Switzerland. In Kippel (Friedl, 1974: 32): 'Wine is drunk mostly at public houses . . . only men patronize these establishments regularly, although women sometimes accompany their husbands on Sunday after church.' Similarly, in rural Hertfordshire Whitehead (1976) found that the pub was a male domain, men spent a good deal of time and money there, and older women supported their segregated culture.

Northern European cities are suffused with beliefs about sex equality and sexual integration that are profoundly shocking to southern Europeans, and even more so to Islamic guestworkers, especially stricter Muslims. The guardianship of women, the value placed on virginity and the segregation of the sexes which the social worker in Lyon (Grillo, 1985) regards as backward in a Tunisian family would be understood by a rural Sicilian man, even though he did not share the Tunisians' faith. Before leaving the honour–shame system it is important to stress the *power* it places in the hands of women.

The position of women in these cultures where the honour–shame system operates is both powerless and extremely powerful. A woman who steps out of line can be, at the extreme, killed, but equally, a woman who steps out of line has destroyed her husband's honour. His fate is in *her* hands.

Underlying the practices about men and women in all the societies of northern and southern Europe are unexamined cosmologies: that is, sets of beliefs about the essential 'nature' of males and females. Anthropologists have been fascinated by these beliefs, and often spend a good deal of time collecting them, especially from men. Before leaving the area of male and female behaviour, a brief summary of the approach is given.

SEXUAL SYMBOLISM

Anthropology since the late 1940s has been much influenced by a theoretical approach called structuralism, which came from France and was popularised in England by Edmund Leach and Mary Douglas. The underlying idea is that all human cultures have world views or cosmologies which depend on binary oppositions. So humans understand their society in terms of oppositions, such as raw *versus* cooked, human *versus* animal, death *versus* life, god *versus* men, and male *versus* female. Many of the cultures of Europe certainly have cosmologies in which the sexes are opposites and danger/pollution/ social chaos come from mixing or blurring sex roles. Pina-Cabral (1986) provides such an analysis for northern Portugal, and the most beautifully written is Bourdieu's (1971) analysis of how male and female are symbolised by the spatial organisation of the Berber house.

Bourdieu starts from a Berber proverb:

> When the proverb says: 'Man is the lamp of the outside and woman the lamp of the inside' it is to be understood that man is the true light, that of the day, and woman the light of the darkness, the dark light; moreover she is, of course, to the moon what man is to the sun.
>
> (1971: 105)

Male and female, light and fire versus darkness and dampness, are then carried forward into the whole arrangement of the house.

The dark and nocturnal, lower part of the house, places of objects that are moist, green or raw – jars of water . . . wood and green fodder – natural place also of beings – oxen and cows, donkeys and mules – and place of natural activities – sleep, the sexual act, giving birth – and the place also of death, is opposed, as nature is to culture, to the light-filled, noble, upper part of the house: this is the place of fire and of objects created by fire – lamp, kitchen utensils, rifle . . . and it is also the place of the two specifically cultural activities that are carried out in the space of the house: cooking and weaving.

(Bourdieu, 1971: 105)

Not everyone accepts such structuralist analyses of belief systems, but for those who *do*, they explain why hostility is aroused by any changes in sex roles. If male v. female is a fundamental division in society, then changes in it are disturbing for members of that society in ways they cannot easily understand.

If European people are uncomfortable when their traditional food and drink is not available, challenges to the patterns of sex roles, with their deeply embedded symbolic loadings, are equally disturbing. If legislation from Brussels about olive oil or sausages is controversial, laws about gender are even more so. Sex segregation or integration, and male domination or sex equality are equally controversial dimensions.

SUGGESTED READING/ACTIVITY

Read Sally Cole's (1991) *Women of the Praia*, the first ethnography of a European fishing community where women went to sea.

Chapter 10

All Babel tongues
Language and identity in Europe

All Babel tongues which flaunt and flow. . .

(Flecker, 1947: 84)

INTRODUCTION

This chapter deals with language in Europe. If there is one issue as deeply personal as food it is language and dialect. The tongues we use are part of our identity, our racial, religious and political sense of self and our gender, our class, our age and our ambitions are embodied and made public in our speech and our writing.

When Henson (1974) wrote a book called *British Social Anthropologists and Language* she was able to subtitle it *A History of Separate Development.* Twenty years later the anthropologists of Europe have made a serious contribution to our understanding of the inter-relationships of language and identity in many parts of Europe. Grillo, for example, has devoted a whole monograph to, and edited a collection of papers on anthropology and the politics of language (Grillo, 1989a, 1989b). There are major monographs on the Breton language movement (McDonald, 1989), on Basque (Urla, 1987; Heiberg, 1989), on Catalan (Woolard, 1989), on Greek (Herzfeld, 1982); and the issues of Gaelic in Ireland and Scotland, of Flemish in Belgium, of Welsh, of Provençal and so on are routinely accepted as legitimate subjects for study. The arrival of guestworkers and immigrants speaking Turkish, Serbo-Croat, Urdu, Bengali, Laotian and Berber has also generated research, especially on education.

Language is also a part of religion: whether the Catholic Church should have abandoned Latin, whether Muslims in Germany should be taught Arabic at government expense, whether Portuguese guestworkers in Denmark should have a Portuguese-speaking priest and if so, who should bear the cost of him, are all language-related issues in modern Europe. When St Bernadette reported that the Virgin Mary had spoken to her in local dialect, not French, or Latin, or Hebrew, or Aramaic, language and religion were being inextricably linked, as they were when the Virgin spoke in Euskera (Basque) at Ezquioga in 1931 (Christian, 1987).

Language is also a political issue. Franco tried to kill Catalan, Basque, Mallorcan and Galician – he wanted everyone to speak Castilian. The Greek junta of 1967–74 tried to outlaw *demotiki* (the normal everyday speech of most Greeks) from official settings such as schools, and return Greece to the use of *Katharevousa*, an élite version of the language which apes ancient Greek. Macedonian is still a 'forbidden' tongue in Greece today.

The language used in schools, and the foundation of schools to teach endangered languages, are also important political issues. Welsh-medium schooling in Wales, the Breton nursery school movement, the Basque schools, the reinstatement of Mallorcan in the schools of Mallorca are all hotly debated.

Accent and dialect are markers of social status. When southern Italians move to the north their accent and dialect mark them out *as* Southerners, and they are stigmatised. In the UK, some accents are high status, others low – and we are judged *by* our accents. In many cultures different modes of speech are appropriate for males and females, for old and young. In some cultures there are ritual forms of language – such as laments for the dead – which are the particular task of women. In other places a man's status may depend on his ability to tell jokes, or engage in verbal duelling, or recount stories.

All these issues are discussed in this chapter, after a brief explanation of how research on language is done. Before addressing the findings of research on language, it is necessary to understand how such data are collected. In this book I have invented two anthropologists, Rachel Verinder and Franklin Blake, doing conventional fieldwork. Rachel would need Castilian Spanish and Galician in her fieldwork, Franklin would need German, and if he decided to study Greek guestworkers in Munich, Greek as well. All researchers have to be sensitive to the languages and dialects that their informants speak, and to the messages that speaking in particular ways carry about them. When Grillo (1985: 18) was trying to establish himself among North African immigrants in Lyon, he tried hanging around the cafés in Place Guichard and Place Gabriel Peri but:

non-Arab customers of such cafes are extremely rare and by and large not welcome, or, rather, treated with great reserve . . . *all* Europeans are regarded with suspicion . . . Fluent knowledge of Arabic . . . is of only marginal help. In fact it can increase suspicion, for who, in France, other than a *pied noir*, a former *colon*, knows Arabic?

Thus having Arabic would be useful in one way, but a problem in another. So while all researchers have to be sensitive to language, and most have to learn one or more 'foreign' tongues, a linguistic project needs a slightly different approach, so let us a imagine a third PhD student, Caroline Ablewhite, setting out from Boarbridge to do a study of bilingualism and language use in Palma, Mallorca. Since the death of Franco, regional languages have become legal, and are even being encouraged. Woolard (1989) is a detailed study of this in Barcelona, so let us imagine that Caroline wants to do something similar to Woolard's research with Mallorcan as her focus. She would go to Palma, find somewhere to live, and then set out to organise some informants for her project. In 1990 the local education system began to advertise for teachers who were interested in learning or resuscitating their Mallorcan so they could, eventually, teach in it rather than Spanish. Caroline could begin by attending the classes for such volunteer teachers, and then she could learn Mallorcan herself, and find a group of enthusiasts. Some would be people who grew up in families speaking the language, others will never have had it and feel robbed of their heritage, some will be hedging their bets in case a grasp of Mallorcan becomes a requirement for holding a teaching job. Those whose parents or grandparents were Mallorcan speakers could introduce Caroline to old people who have always spoken the language. Those who feel 'robbed' will probably be in touch with enthusiasts for the restoration of regional languages, and can help Caroline meet them. The 'bet-hedgers' may be hostile to Mallorcan, and would provide a pro-Castilian Spanish group for her to interview.

Once Caroline has found some people who have Mallorcan, she can begin to use classic socio-linguistic research techniques. These might include observing when, where and to whom her informants spoke Mallorcan and when, where and to whom Castilian; conducting a matched-guise test (explained below) in secondary schools; doing a content analysis of official documents, political speeches, addresses at ceremonies and so on; and/or observing the interaction patterns in Mallorcan classes. The matched-guise test is often used in socio-linguistic research: typically a researcher gets two or three bilingual speakers to read the same passage in each language, plays the tapes to schoolchildren, and asks them to rate the speakers as more or less honest, reliable, proud, posh, snobbish, likeable, progressive, intelligent, generous, happy and so on. People are willing to impute all kinds of qualities to a speaker merely on their accent, dialect and language: for example, when people in England hear a woman speak standard (BBC) English she will be rated more competent, more feminine and more capable of doing a man's job than the same woman heard speaking with a regional accent such as Liverpudlian or cockney (Elyan *et al.*, 1978). So, our hypothetical researcher could discover how adolescents at school in Palma judge Mallorcan speakers compared to Castilian speakers (or Catalan speakers – because Mallorcan can be seen as a regional dialect of Catalan so a Mallorcan/Catalan/Castilian judgement might be particularly interesting). After her fifteen months in Palma, Caroline should know a good deal about whether Mallorcan is going to come back as one of the languages in Palma, and if so whether it will be a 'family' language, or a public one or both.

THE MANY LANGUAGES IN EUROPE

Very few countries, regions, cities, towns, communities or even villages in Europe are inhabited by people who all share one language. Many countries are officially bilingual, with all government documents, all public notices and all educational establishments working in both. In Belgium, which is also an officially bilingual country, the two languages, French and Flemish, are dominant in two regions, and 'overlap' in Brussels. In Finland, for example, Swedish is an official language and notices in post offices and on buses are in both Finnish and Swedish. The universities teach in both languages, and books are published and sold in both. Swedish is a legacy of the time when Finland was a Swedish 'colony' and it is the old élite who speak and write it today. Thus a famous professor of history like Matti Klinge (1981) is fully bilingual, but teaches in Swedish and often speaks it from choice. A bus driver or a canteen worker may not have any fluency in Swedish and would choose to speak Finnish all the time, and a

Greek guestworker would probably not bother to learn Swedish at all. Here the two official languages are mainly markers of 'class'.

INDIGENOUS LANGUAGE MINORITIES

Many European countries have linguistic minorities who have been there for centuries: as the United Kingdom has Welsh speakers and Scots Gaelic speakers so France has Breton speakers and in the north-east of Italy there are people who speak German and so on. The area of Germany near Stuttgart when Spindler (1973) studied the village of Burbach was Schwabisch-speaking rather than High German-speaking.

> Within the family, within the schools, within the peer group, at the taverns, the use of Schwabisch is recognised as a membership card in the native community, the community that belongs.
> (p. 19)

This is not just a difference of dialect.

> There is a Schwabisch culture and character as well as a language. There are songs and jokes, pride in the slowmoving, thoughtful, shrewd character of 'die dummen Schwaben'.
> (p. 19)

Schwabisch is an old-established language in that region, which pre-dates by centuries the political existence of 'Germany'. Many other countries have pockets of people using minority languages. When Boissevain went to Malta in 1960 the use of Maltese and English was significant of both social class and level of intimacy. The type of Maltese spoken also varied between town and country.

> There is a noticeable difference between the heavy consonants and broad vowels of the uneducated countryman, and the English-accented Maltese of the inhabitants of the Sliema, many of whose children speak more English than Maltese. There are also differences in vocabulary and inflection, for the language spoken in Valletta and the towns contains many more Italian and English words and expressions than the village Maltese.
> (Boissevain, 1965: 28)

The schools taught a standardised form of Maltese, *il-Malti bil-pulit*, which all children were encouraged to speak. When Boissevain was preparing to do his fieldwork in London he had Maltese lessons from a teacher there but: 'Francis Chetcuti, in common with all educated Maltese, found it difficult to speak Maltese with a non-Maltese' (1980: 104). This is typical of many countries where a language may be a mark of intimacy and belonging to an in-group, or of rustic status, or of sophisticated urbanese.

Minority languages may be dying, or struggling for survival, or booming. When Brogger (1971) studied Montevarese, a south Italian town, the older people spoke Greek, but the younger ones thought this was old-fashioned and preferred Italian. Greek had been the language of that area since it was part of the Byzantine empire a thousand years before, long before 'Italy' existed.

Some countries have policies of encouraging such minority languages, others have tried to suppress them or outlaw them, others have no policy at all. The Republic of Ireland has had a campaign to keep Gaelic alive in the *Gaeltacht* (the heartland) since 1893 when the Gaelic League was founded. The Catholic Church in Ireland has a union of Gaelic speaking priests (*Cumann na Sagait*) and since the Second Vatican Council they have revived the Gaelic mass, and encouraged piety and the language together. The government of the Republic has a policy of recognising certain communities as Irish-speaking (*Gaeltacht*) and giving grants and subsidies to them. The language is taught in the schools, and there are prizes for communities that promote the use of the language. Scheper-Hughes (1979: 60-61) is sceptical of these policies, and concludes:

> the Irish language was already moribund at the time the language movement began, and persistent efforts to preserve it in the isolated Blasket and Aran islands or to revive it in semi-isolated coastal areas like Ballybran have been largely unsuccessful.
>
> (p. 59)

Messenger (1969) makes the same point about Inis Beag where Irish was rejected by the locals.

The future of the Welsh language in Wales is equally problematic. Strong feelings are aroused by all discussions of the Welsh language, mass media in Wales and Welsh language teaching. The research and its context is described in some detail because it is a topic on which I have written elsewhere (Delamont, 1987). In February 1987 *The Times Educational Supplement* (*TES*) carried a short piece in its 'Talkback' section – where personal, idiosyncratic opinions can be expressed – by Tim Williams (1987). The author was described by the *TES* as an employee of the National Union of Teachers (NUT) who was working on a PhD thesis on the anglicisation of Wales. Williams claimed that Welsh-medium schooling, and the teaching of Welsh in English-medium schools, were, at best, a waste of money and, at worst, harming the life chances of working-class children. In passing, Williams attacked proponents of Welsh, and Welsh language media: 'The Welsh-language lobby has powerful friends and few enemies. A stifling consensus has emerged which prevents awkward questions being raised, let alone answered' (Williams, 1987: 20).

The three letters published in response (*TES* 20 March 1987) included a parent who described Welsh-medium schooling as a 'dubious human experiment', and an NUT official who accused Williams of being inconsistent, disingenuous and ignorant of the research on bilingual schooling. Fred Jarvis, the General Secretary of the NUT, wrote to disown Williams and disassociate the Union from the position he had taken. Such is the climate in which any research carried out on schooling in Welsh, the state of the language and the Welsh-language television channel (S4C) is received.

English language media are routinely seen as a major source of pressure on the minority languages of Britain. Mackinnon writing about Gaelic in Barra and Harris says:

> The principal anglicising forces at work in these communities can be seen as originating from outwith. Such are the use of English as an official language, economic pressures promoting migration, an intrusive educational system *and mass media* . . .
>
> (1987a: 23; emphasis mine)

Evans (1982: 3) petitioning the Home Secretary to get S4C established wrote:

> The good we feel that is being done in the nursery and primary schools in teaching the Welsh language to our children is being counteracted and eroded by the amount of English language TV being shown.

Similar arguments about the language of the capital eroding minority languages at the peripheries can be found elsewhere in Europe. Woolard (1988) suggests for example, that Castilian mass media are one form of cultural hegemony operating to undermine Catalan.

Television and radio broadcasts from London are primarily blamed for the anglicisation of Wales and Scotland, but newspapers, magazines, pop music and the cinema are also accused of disseminating both British and American English, and their accompanying cultural systems. Television is the focus of most research attention and public debate, but the other media are briefly discussed. Advocates of the survival and revival of the Welsh language became increasingly concerned about the anglicising power of television in the period after the 1950s, and pressure built up for a Welsh-language TV channel. After 1974 serious campaigning began which led, after the threatened hunger strike of Gwynfor Evans, to S4C.

The campaign for S4C, with the slogan '*Yr Unig Ateb*' (the only answer), drew its strength from a deep unease about the power of television. Research on how far S4C is reaching its potential audience and what, if any, impact it is having on Welsh life and language is controversial. The experiences of McDonald (1987), when her historical and ethnographic work on Breton was published and immediately became engulfed in the ongoing fierce controversies about the past and future of Breton language and culture, are a salutary lesson for social scientists examining Welsh and Welsh media.

Since the launch of S4C Williams and Thomas (1985) have conducted the government's research on the impact of S4C on the Welsh language, while Peter Wynne Thomas (1986, 1987) questioned 6,000 children in Welsh-medium schools about their media use. Williams and Thomas conducted three linked pieces of research. There was a national survey to discover whether S4C was being viewed and how it was valued; a study of how the Welsh language is changing; and some preliminary work on whether S4C is introducing Welsh speakers to a form of 'Received Pronunciation' or 'Standard Welsh'. All three parts of the study were done on small numbers of respondents.

The national survey used a sample of 108 people who could speak Welsh, representing both sexes, the age range 20–70, and all social classes, who were located in twelve communities spread throughout Wales in areas of high, medium and low density of Welsh-speaking. These people were asked about their viewing and listening patterns and about their use of Welsh in a variety of contexts or domains: family, religion, education, bureaucratic, work, community and among peers. When discussing the use of Welsh in different domains Williams and Thomas (1985: 25) make the important point that S4C might not increase the *number* of

Welsh speakers, but might widen the size and domains in which Welsh speakers use the language. The 108 respondents reported that they preferred their religious programmes in Welsh, and also that soap operas, quizzes and musical shows were better in Welsh than in English. Also, they implied that they watched Welsh programmes even when they felt the English version of the same programme type was 'better'.

Grammar, pronunciation and vocabulary were the focus of the second part of the investigation: the community studies. Although Williams and Thomas label this approach participant observation, the data gathering was based on one interview, rather than long-term residence in the communities with detailed observation. Data were gathered in Merthyr Tydfil and the surrounding catchment area of Rhydfelen School (a pioneer Welsh-medium secondary school near Pontypridd), and in Aberdaron in Gwynedd, part of the heartland of Welsh language and culture. The analysis showed a 'generation gap', in that children spoke in ways different from their parents. Children's Welsh language use showed smaller percentages of the 'correct' form than that of adults. However, children of non-Welsh-speaking parents use the 'correct' forms more frequently than pupils from Welsh-speaking homes on most of the 'test' words used by the researchers.

The final aspect of Williams' and Thomas's study was a classic 'matched guise' experiment conducted on thirty-two respondents in the Vale of Conwy. A 'matched guise' experiment involves getting an actress to record the same passage in two or more dialects. These are played to subjects, who are not aware that all the voices are one actor's, and the subjects are asked to rate the 'speakers' as 'intelligent', 'ambitious', 'masculine', 'posh' or whatever. The Bangor team used one formal, broadcasting voice and five dialect forms, including one representing a 'learner'. As we might expect the 'voice' of S4C was rated as 'upper middle class' rather than working-class, as was the 'learner'. The 'S4C' voice was also rated as the most trustworthy, reliable and authoritative. The 'learner' was seen as untrustworthy and cold. The voice which was closest to the dialect of the Vale of Conwy was judged to be that of a speaker from a working-class background, who lacked authority but would be a good workmate and an empathetic friend. Overall then, the S4C voice and the 'learner's voice' were seen as socially distant from the judges rather than neighbourly.

Peter Wynne Thomas's (1986, 1987) follow-up of the media preferences of pupils in Welsh-medium secondary schools provides data on a much larger sample. Thomas issued 6,000 questionnaires to Welsh-speaking adolescents throughout Wales and found different patterns of Welsh TV viewing between pupils whose parents were monoglot English and those from Welsh-speaking homes where the language is and is not used between the members. Adolescents in North Wales were more likely to come from homes where both parents habitually speak Welsh, whereas 44 per cent of those in south-east Wales had no Welsh spoken in their homes. There are, however, some children whose parents can speak Welsh, but choose not to do so. These teenagers are the least likely to watch S4C – less likely than their schoolfellows from families where the parents cannot speak Welsh.

The pupils from Welsh-speaking homes reported that they also used Welsh in their neighbourhood and community (i.e. to local shopkeepers), and this was less common among those from homes where Welsh is known but unused, or not known. However, *all* the teenagers told Thomas that they used Welsh to their schoolfellows and teachers. He concludes: 'the school is to some measure succeeding in providing the necessary environment for fostering the *voluntary* use of Welsh by young teenagers' (1986: 319).

Peter Wynne Thomas is therefore optimistic that S4C and Welsh medium schooling are helping 'save' Welsh, a much more positive conclusion than Scheper-Hughes's (1979) on Ireland, or McDonald's (1989) on Breton, which is discussed later in the chapter. Heiberg (1989) and Woolard (1989) are optimistic about Basque and Catalan surviving, Chapman (1992) and McDonald (1989) are pessimistic about Breton, just as Chapman (1978) and Mewett (1982a: 226) are pessimistic about Gaelic in Scotland.

What *is* clear about the survival or loss of such indigenous minority languages is that researchers who conclude that a language is dying despite schools or mass media in the language are reviled (see McDonald, 1987). Equally controversial are studies of language and new linguistic minorities, such as Turkish Cypriots in London, Serbian guestworkers in Berlin or Algerians in Lyon.

THE EDUCATION OF 'IMMIGRANT' CHILDREN

The arrival of guestworkers, immigrants and refugees in European countries produces problems for the education system. In the area of London which was served by the Inner London Education Authority (ILEA) there were 187 different mother-tongues *known*

to be in the schools (Rosen and Burgess, 1980). A city like Cardiff
– with a population of a quarter of a million – has at least eighty
mother-tongues. The Linguistic Minorities Project (1985) did a
survey in Coventry, Bradford, and two London boroughs, focused
on speakers of Portuguese, Italian, Turkish, Greek, Gujerati,
'Chinese' (a heading covering several very different languages),
Bengali, Punjabi and Polish. These were the languages which had
a large number of speakers who could be traced for study. Any
other northern European city would easily generate that many
languages, though not the same ones, because the pattern
depends on which refugees, immigrants, guestworkers and so on
have settled there (e.g. Brunt, 1989 on Utrecht).

Camilleri (1986) discussed the educational problems such
linguistic minorities pose for the school systems of northern Europe,
and Grillo (1989a) is a thorough account of how France and Great
Britain have faced up to educating 'immigrant' children (see also
Eldering and Kloprogge, 1989). There are diametrically opposed
views among both scholars who understand the issues and ordinary
people who do not about what are the best ways to educate children
whose home language (mother-tongue) is not English. None of the
northern European countries has succeeded yet in designing an
education system which produces academically successful 18- or
19-year-olds from the immigrant and guestworker communities in
sufficient numbers: too many German Turks, Belgian Greeks, French
Moroccans and British Bangladeshi are not getting the education
they deserve. The papers collected by Wilpert (1988a) focus on this
problem in Belgium (Bastenier and Dassetto, 1988), Germany
(Wilpert 1988b), France (Palidda and Minoz, 1988), the UK (Cross,
1988) and Switzerland (Fibbi and Rham, 1988). The northern
European countries need to solve this problem.

At the heart of the debate is a disagreement. Is it better to start
children off in their mother-tongue, get them literate and feeling
positive about schooling and gradually switch them to the majority
tongue of the 'host' country (Danish, Dutch, French or whatever)
or should all schooling be in the language of the host nation from
the outset? Some commentators take political or moral positions
on this, but it should be decided on the basis of research.
Countries should adopt the pattern which maximises the achieve-
ments of children over their school careers. Unfortunately the
research is mostly American, so may not apply in Europe, and is
inconclusive (see *Educational Researcher*, March 1992). Until it is

clear which system is best, the arguments will certainly rage. (As language is such a controversial and emotional issue, even clear-cut research findings will not stop the arguments.) Providing mother-tongue teaching is also complicated when there are many different minorities in a town. If all the guestworker children in one town are Turkish-speaking the issue is much simpler than a city with 187 different mother-tongues.

Just as problematic as the appropriate language for the education of 'immigrant' children is the topic of language and gender.

LANGUAGE AND GENDER

There are three main aspects of language and gender to be discussed in this section: the idea of 'genderlects' in majority languages, those forms of language, such as mourning laments, which are only appropriate for one sex or the other, and the evidence on women's roles and men's roles in perpetuating or killing minority languages.

Researchers on language have been interested in whether men and women speak differently for the past twenty years. It transpires that many languages have 'genderlects': that is, men and women use different vocabularies, grammatical structures and intonation patterns. Graddol and Swann (1989) is an introduction to this research, while Tannen (1991) is a much publicised study of men's and women's language use in the USA. Graddol and Swann (1989: 119–124) deal with French, German and English, so it is a good place to start further reading on the topic, which is not explored here. The whole topic of genderlects becomes particularly important when the survival or death of a minority language is under consideration, but does also have an impact on majority languages. In English, for example, women are more likely to speak 'correct' English rather than the local dialects, than men of the same class and education level. It appears that speaking 'nicely' is part of being respectable, ladylike and feminine.

Research on particular forms of language, especially ritual forms, has been done in many European countries. Scholars have been keen to collect mourning laments, which are often the domain of women. The most dramatic are the *miroloyia* (words of destiny), of the Mani, the desolate peninsula in the south of mainland Greece. They are improvised around certain set phrases, in sixteen-syllable couplets and some women become famous *miroloyistrias.* The Fermors (1958: 61) were in Areopolis and told a friend, George, they had never heard a full lament. The friend immediately swept them off to meet his cousin Eleni

> one of the last *miroloyistrias* in the Deep Mani . . . his old aunt and his cousin Eleni were knitting under a pomegranate tree. His cousin was a handsome, plump young woman with apple-cheeks, quite unlike the sombre crone I had expected.

Initially Eleni refused to sing, because there had not been a death, but finally she was persuaded to sing the *miroloy* composed for a British pilot shot down at Limeni during the Second World War. George explained: 'We gave him a fine funeral and Eleni sang the miroloy: we were all very sorry for him' (Fermor, 1958: 61–62). Fermor was mesmerised, managed to record it, and presents it in translation in his book. In translation it includes:

> His bravery lays us deep in his debt,
> For it was for the honour of Greece that he came
> What will his mother and sisters do without him?

These are classic elements: praise for the dead and rhetorical questions about the fate of those left behind. Seremetakis (1991) and Caraveli (1980) have researched such laments. Seremetakis (1991) contains two *miroloi* sung by a woman called Kalliopi fifty years apart. In 1932 Kalliopi, a teacher, became engaged to a young male teacher but before they could marry he died of tuberculosis. Kalliopi's *miroloy* from 1932 was recalled for Seremetakis in 1983 by her niece, another female relative, and Kalliopi herself. In 1984 Kalliopi's husband – to whom she had been married in 1934, died, and Seremetakis also collected her lament for Panayiotis. The two make an interesting contrast (1991: 130–143). Kalliopi is described as having 'the *miroloi* innate in her' (130) and it is clear that a woman's status in the community is heightened by skill at composition. As Fermor says:

> For death and burial are one of the few occasions in Greek peasant life when women come into their own and take over. After long years of drudgery and silence and being told to shut up they are suddenly on top and there is no doubt that for some of the them, famous *miroloyistrias*, wailers with a turn for acting and a gift of improvisation, these are moments secretly longed for . . . Some of them are in great demand.

> (1958: 57)

A linguistic phenomenon among men which has equally capti-
vated researchers is competitive verse making or insult swapping.
This has been reported from several cultures. In highland Corsica
(Simon, 1976) men competed for status in speech competitions;
verses had to be improvised in a duel, each man trying to cap the
verse of his opponent until one was outwitted. In the mountains of
Crete men get status from composing *mantinadies*. Fermor (1958:
58) who spent part of the war in the Cretan mountains with the
resistance, comments on 'the speed with which the Cretans can
turn any incident on the spot into a faultless rhyming couplet and
each time with an epigrammatic sting in the second line'. Herzfeld
(1985) is the academic volume on these hardy shepherds and their
competitive masculinity. Caraveli (1985) is an account of *mantinadies* on Karpathos.

Apart from such dramatic and competitive gender-specific uses
of language, there are several studies in 'bilingual' communities
which show gender differences in the use of the two languages.
Some of the most careful fieldwork on this has been done in
Brittany, where a female researcher (McDonald, 1989) and a male
(Chapman, 1992) have both gathered data. Chapman summarises
the complexity of language use in Plouturiec.

> Everybody is a fluent French speaker; most people over 40 *can*
> speak Breton and many do in normal daily life; no children or
> teenagers speak Breton; for those who are bilingual, French and
> Breton serve different social functions.
>
> (1992: 41–42)

Chapman tried to do his fieldwork by pretending to be an English-
speaker who did not speak French and so would only learn Breton.
However, this did not work. It was 'normal' for a man, of his age and
obviously educated, *not* to speak Breton at all. People in Plouturiec
found his desire to learn Breton baffling, and if he had not admitted
to having French they would have 'thought I was truly mad' (p. 45).
The pattern of languages for a young man is as follows:

> A young man who speaks French and understands Breton . . . is
> normal. One who speaks French and does not understand
> Breton is also normal. One who speaks French and wishes to
> learn Breton is weird. One who does not speak French and
> wishes to learn only Breton is a kind of unimaginable
> nightmare.

Chapman was 28, and so 'Breton was not appropriate for me' (p. 46). McDonald (1989: 243-255) contains a description of how gender and language interact in rural areas: 'Women can define their femininity, and men their masculinity, through the language they use' (p. 247). Men, when with other men of the same age in settings such as bars and the fields, speak Breton, because to speak French would be 'putting on airs'. Women who work in the fields may speak both Breton and French, and will speak Breton with their husbands, *but* when with other women, especially in the 'clean' front room, French is used to emphasise how feminine, ladylike and urbane they all are.

> When the men are present at evening gatherings of the whole village, such as occurs at New Year, the women sit together at one end of a long table with their sweet cakes and sweet drinks and speak predominantly French, and the men pack together at the other end in a haze of cigarette smoke, eating cheap *pâté*, drinking hard liquor, playing dominoes or cards, and speaking predominantly Breton.
>
> (McDonald, 1989: 248)

Into that pattern come outsiders who are enthusiastic about recycling, living off the land, and reinvigorating Breton. These outsiders reject the 'femininity' of local women, and also the association of French with being ladylike. McDonald gives a fascinating account of the complexities of when men and women speak Breton, if they have ever learnt it, and when they do not.

Insofar as women are primarily responsible for rearing small children, whether or not children learn minority languages such as Schwabisch, Breton, Welsh or Scots Gaelic will be very dependent on *women's* attitudes to the language. If women do not pass a minority language on to the children, its chances of survival are slim.

Several of the types of language associated with only men or only women are related to religious behaviour. Only men can be Catholic and Greek Orthodox priests, so only males should speak the priests' words in the divine service. Only men can be imams in the mosque and only men should read the Koran in public. The funeral laments of the Mani are a 'religious' language used by women.

There are also ways in which religion is related to minority languages. McDonald (1989: 244–245) reports on the use of Breton at the old abbey of Le Reliq, and at Ploune'our a new priest who arrived in 1981 used Breton hymns in the weekly mass, plus the old Latin *credo*. The locals enjoyed these language changes from French, but did *not* want sermons in Breton, for as the priest told McDonald, it carried the smell of cow dung: that is, reminded them of a peasant way of life the parishioners had proudly left behind.

Language is, therefore, another way in which identity is maintained, asserted and reproduced. It is no accident that many of the contributors to Sharon MacDonald's (1993) edited collection, *Inside European Identities*, deal with language: with language choices, rights to tell stories, and demands to learn 'traditional' tongues.

SUGGESTED READING/ACTIVITY

Read A. Caraveli (1982) 'The song beyond the song' for a moving account of a gender-specific speech pattern.

Chapter 11

Ringed with a lake of fire
Conclusions

> the hidden sun
> That rings black Cyprus with a lake of fire. . .
>
> (Flecker, 1947: 138)

The lake of fire is, of course, the sea round Cyprus ablaze in the setting sun. My intention in the book has been to inspire my readers to plunge into that lake of fire: to immerse themselves in the anthropological literature on Europe. Whether the reader turns to an account of life in a Danish village in the 1950s (Anderson and Anderson, 1964), or to the impact of a nuclear power station on a Breton community (Zonabend, 1993), the fascination of the anthropological monograph should now be apparent. I hope that the readers will turn to Holmes's (1989) study of worker peasants in Friuli and to Cowan's (1990) study of dance in northern Greece before they go on holiday to Venice or Thessaloniki or set off for their 'year abroad' in Italy or Greece.

Anthropology has been a small, élite discipline, located in a minority of British universities, with few 'outreach' courses for students in other disciplines. My intention has been to provide a way into the discipline for student outsiders who, I hope will share my enthusiasms for the lake of fire. I hope, also that I have shown the relevance of social anthropological studies to the contemporary world and to urban living. A villager told Harriet Rosenberg that the changed ecology of the Alpine valley was symbolised by the vanished eagle: 'Today we see no eagles soaring over the mountains of Abriès . . . we have no more eagles (Rosenberg, 1988: 211). Anthropology can illuminate life after the eagle has vanished.

Glossary of anthropological terms

There are some technical anthropological terms you may come across in articles and books.

Participant observation/fieldwork/ethnography refers to how anthropologists get their data.

The *nuclear family* is a man, woman and their children. The *extended family* is a three-generation family, and/or family of several cousins/second cousins, etc.

Many societies distinguish between two types of cousin: *cross-cousins* are the chidren of your father's sister(s) and your mother's brother(s). *Parallel cousins* are the children of your father's brother(s) and your mother's sister(s). In some societies you are allowed to marry cross-cousins but *not* parallel cousins.

Uxorilocal residence means once a couple marry they live near or with the wife's family. The opposite is virilocal – living near the husband's family. This matters a great deal in some cultures.

It is also important to distinguish *bridewealth* from dowry – a *dowry* is the wealth (a house, money, linens, cattle, a boat . . .) a woman brings to the marriage. Bridewealth (*not* found in Europe) is where the groom has to 'buy' his bride from her family with money/cattle/goats or something.

Affines are your relatives by marriage (in-laws).

Agnatic kin are those related to you through your father.

Things to do with marriage have *-gamy* at the end. *Endogamy* means marrying *inside* a boundary – i.e. marrying someone from the same village, or the same religion or language group. *Exogamy* is marrying 'out' – i.e. choosing a spouse from a different village, tribe or language group.

Directory of research sites

This is an alphabetical list of the field sites, country by country, mentioned in the book. Most of the names, especially of small places, are pseudonyms chosen by the researcher to protect the real people s/he studied. It is noticeable that occasionally two researchers have chosen the same pseudonym for a different site, and that sometimes researchers used a pseudonym in their early writing and then the 'real' name later.

AUSTRIA

Sankt Martin – in the Austrian Tyrol, a mountain farming community of 1020 studied by Heppenstall (1971).
Wiener Neustadt – nearest town to the village studied by Thornton (1987).

BELGIUM

Château-Gérard – village in the old Principality, or modern Land of Liège, in the Walloon (French-speaking) part of Belgium. Studied by Turney-High (1953).

CYPRUS

Alona – village in the Pitsilia area of the Troodos mountains studied by Peristiany (1966a).
Argaki – real name of village in Cyprus now occupied by the Turks, originally a Greek Cypriot village studied by Loizos (1975).
Kaio – pseudonym of Argaki (see above).

Pitsilia – area in the Troodos Mountains studied by Peristiany (1966a).

FRANCE

Abriès – a village in the Hautes-Alpes with a population of 200 when studied by Rosenberg (1988).

Auguste – county town of a commune in the Pyrenees with 320 permanent inhabitants, studied by Blaxter (1971).

Auxerre – chief town of the Yonne (see below).

Bocage – deliberately vague term used by Favret-Saada (1980) to protect informants in her study of rural witchcraft beliefs – it means 'country of high hedges'.

Chanzeaux – village in Anjou, France, studied by Wylie with a team of students (1957).

Colpied – a low mountain village in the Basse-Alpes department of France studied by Rayna Rapp Reiter (1972).

Grand Frault – a community in north-eastern France studied by Rogers (1985).

Houat – village on an island off the coast of Brittany studied by Jorion (1977).

La Feuillée – a small, inland community in Brittany studied by Badone (1990).

La Roche – set of hamlets in the Basse-Alpes, only 10 miles from Italy. Population 200. Studied by Rosenberg, Reiter and Reiter (1973).

Lourdes – real name of major French pilgrimage site. Studied by Marnham (1980) Turner and Turner (1978), Dahlberg (1991) and Eade (1991).

Lyon – real name of a city in central France where Grillo (1985) studied immigration.

Melize – village in Hautes-Alpes with population of 190. Ski-ing resort. Researched by Rosenberg, Reiter and Reiter (1973).

Minot – village in Burgundy where Zonabend (1984) did oral history.

Montagnac – real name of Colpied. When revisisted in 1980 had a population of 180 residents and 400 summer vacationers (Rapp, 1986).

Montaillou – village where inquisition investigated Cathars between 1294-1324. Site of famous historical work by Ladurie (1975).

Pellaport – village of 250 people in the northern French Jura. A dairying community studied by Layton (1971).

Peyrane – village in Avignon region of southern France, where Provençal is spoken. Samuel Beckett spent the war there. Studied by Wylie (1957).

Pinellu – mountain village in Corsica studied by Simon (1976). Population of 180 in 1970.

Plodemet – village in Brittany, France, studied by Morin (1971).

Plouguerneau – a coastal, tourist area of Brittany studied by Badone (1990).

Plouneour – a commune of twenty-seven villages in rural Finistère, Brittany. One village here, Menez, was studied by McDonald (1989).

Plozevet – village in Brittany, France, studied by Burguière (1977) Real name of Plodemet.

Poitiers – real name of French city where Boisvert (1987) studied Portugese immigrants.

Pont l'Abbé – Breton community near Quimper, centre of 'lost' Breton culture lamented by Helias (1978).

Quarré-les-Tombes – small market town in the Yonne (see below).

Rennes – real name of city in Brittany where McDonald (1989) did research.

Roussillon – real name of Peyrane (see above).

Sainte-Engrâce – Basque mountain community studied by Ott (1981).

Sainte-Marie-de-la-Mer – French pilgrimage site with a black Virgin (Sara), a place of pilgrimage for gypsies (Quintana and Floyd, 1972).

Saint Martin de Londres – near Montpelier, an area where shepherds decorate their sheep with dyed tufts on their backs before moving them on the six-day trek to the other side of the Cevennes.

St Veran – home of the park-keeper peasants studied by Franklin (1969).

Saint-Jean-Trolimen – a parish in Brittany studied by Segalen (1991).

Ste Foy – a rural community in south-western France studied by Rogers (1985). In Aveyron, in the Langue d'Oc area, Roquefort cheese is the main product.

Strasbourg – actual name of city on the French/German border (in the Alsace region) studied by Gaines (1985).

Valloire – John and Susan Hutson (1971) used this as the pseudo-nym of a village in the Alps near the Italian border. Since the 1950s it had been developed as a ski-resort. Villepontoux (1981) used this pseudonym for a village in the Maurienne.

Wissous – 'suburb' of Paris studied by R.T. and B.G. Anderson (1962).

Yonne – a department in the Burgundy region of France studied by Abeles (1991).

GERMANY

Burgbach – village near Stuttgart, Germany studied by George and Louise Spindler, see Spindler (1973).

Hausen – a town in Germany where Yucel (1987) studied Turkish businessmen.

Hohenlohe-Franken – area in south-west Germany where Golde (1975) studied two farming villages.

Neuss – real name of town in West Germany which was main migration destination of emigrants from Alcudia de la Guadix, studied by Rhoades (1979a).

Nordstadt – industrial town with traditional glass-blowing industry. Guestworkers were studied by Sontz (1987).

Offenbach – town in Germany where Yucel (1987) studied Turkish guestworkers.

Rheinstadt – town with factories where Cari, a Spanish woman studied by Goodman (1987), worked in a sweet factory.

Schonhausen – community near Stuttgart, Germany, studied by the Spindlers (1987).

GREECE

Ambeli – tiny hamlet in Euboea (Evia), the large island in Greece studied by du Boulay (1974).

Ammouliani – village on islands off Chalkidhiki with 450 inhabit-ants studied by Salamone (1986).

Amorgos – real name of small Greek island studied by Connell (1980).

Apeiranthos – a village on the Greek island of Naxos studied by Stewart (1991).

Asi Gonia – a village in western Crete with transhumant herders and olive growers studied by Machin (1983).

Ayia Eleni – town in Serres in Macedonia, Greece famous for the *Anastenarides* (fire walkers) studied by Danforth (1989).

Glendi – a village in the mountains of Crete, Greece, studied by Herzfeld (1985).

Karpofora – mainland village studied by Aschenbrenner (1986).

Nafplion – a real town in the Peloponnese studied by Zinovieff (1991a).

Nea Ephesus – suburb on former open land north-east of Piraeus harbour built to take refugees in 1922. In 1971 there were 86,000 people there. Studied by Hirschon (1989).

Nisi – Aegean island with population of 750, studied by Dioniso-poulos-Mass (1976).

Nisos – a tiny island in the Aegean sea studied by Kenna (1976).

Pefko – a village on Rhodes studied by Herzfeld (1980).

Platanos – a mainland Greek town with a tourist trade studied by Zinovieff (1991a).

Psilafi – village in Crete, Greece, studied by Makris (1992).

Rethemno – real name of town in Crete, Greece, studied by Herzfeld (1991).

Sohos – a town in central Macedonia, Greece, studied by Cowan (1990).

Spartohori – a village on the tiny island of Meganisi studied by Just (1991).

Tinos – real name of Greek island with famous icon of the *Panayia*, studied by Dubisch (1986).

Yerania – area of 1922 refugee settlement near Piraeus studied by Hirschon (1983).

ITALY

Accettura – Italian town studied by Colclough (1971).

Agnone – town in the Molise, in a high valley studied by Douglass (1980). Population down to 6,966 by 1920 from 11,615 in 1877.

Albora – a *quartiere* outside the old city of Bologna, in northern Italy, studied by Kertzer (1980).

Ascioli Piceno – a city north of Rome, Italy, in the region of Le Marche studied by Romanucci-Ross (1991).

Bari – port and town in the south-east of Italy where Fiat built a factory studied by Amin (1985).

Baronessa – a *latifondo* (great estate) in Sicily, used as a case study by Blok (1974).

Basilicata – area surrounding the agrotown studied by Cornelisen (1976).

Bassano – a town of 40,000 people in the Veneto region of northern Italy studied by Filippucci (1992).

Bosa – a Sardinian agrotown studied by Counihan (1985).

Brazzano – village in the Friuli where in the sixteenth century people believed in the *benandanti* (see Ginzburg, 1983).

Calimera – village studied by Maraspini (1968).

Colleverde – small commune in Perugia studied by Silverman (1977).

Colombaio – village in the hills of central Italy with a population of 700, studied by Wade (1971).

Eboli – symbolic boundary of central Italy for the inhabitants of Gagliano (see below) in the 1930s. They told Levi (1982) 'Christ stopped at Eboli', meaning that the *mezzogiorno* started south of Eboli.

Franza – village studied by Lopreato (1967).

Gagliano – town in Lucania where Carlo Levi (1982) was exiled by Mussolini in the 1930s.

Garre – Sicilian town studied by Giovannini (1986).

Genuardo – Sicilan rural area where Blok (1974) conducted a study of the history of the mafia. In mountains of western Sicily near Palermo.

Iassico – village in the Friuli where Paolo Gasparutto, the famous night battler (*benandante*) lived, whose interrogation by the inquisi tion in 1575 is reconstructed by Ginzburg (1983).

Lamie di Olimpia – hamlet in southern Italy used as base for Galt's (1991) research on the Locorotondo (see below).

Lecce – real name of city in southern Italy, from which agricultural workers were hired to get in the tobacco crop to Pisticci (see below).

Leverano – village near Lecce, population 13,028 studied by King, Strachan and Mortimer (1986).

Losa – 800 people live in this community on the northern edge of the Maritime Alps, studied by Bailey (1971c).

Luco – agrotown in the Abruzzi region of Italy studied by White (1980).

Malva – a village near Ascoli Piceno in Italy studied by Romanucci-Ross (1991).

Matera – town in the south of Italy where the poorest families lived in caves until the 1950s. Researched by Tentori (1976).

Milocca – village in Sicily studied by Gower Chapman (1971) in the 1920s and 1930s.

Montecastello di Vibio – a town of 350 inhabitants in the Tiber Valley, central Italy, studied by Silverman (1975).

Montegrano – agrotown studied by Banfield (1958), in the province of Potenza with population of 3,400.

Montelaterone – a Tuscan village in Italy studied by Pratt (1984).

Montevarese – southern Italian agrotown where Greek was the local language as late as the 1950s studied by Brogger (1971).

Murgia dei Trulli – the Plateau of the Trulli in a zone of Apulia, studied by Galt (1991).

Naples – Italian city researched by Belmonte (1979), Pardo (1989), Allum (1973) and Chubb (1982).

Ollolai – Sardinian sheep-rearing village studied by Berger (1986).

Palermo – real name of the capital of the Italian island of Sicily studied by Cucchiari (1988).

Pantellaria – tiny Italian island off the coast of Sicily studied by Galt (1982).

Pertosa – hill-top village in the central Apennine uplands of central Italy studied by Colclough (1971).

Pisticci – agrotown in southern Italy studied by Davis (1973).

Rubignacco – one of the seven outlying rural settlements in the commune of Cividale de Friuli, in the north-east of Italy near Venice. There were 100 families there when studied by Holmes (1983).

San Giovanni Rotondo – town in the heel of Italy where Padre Pío – a candidate for sainthood – lived till his death in 1968. Studied by McKevitt (1991).

Siena – real name of northern Italian city famous for the *Palio*, a 'medieval' religious horse race. Studied by Park (1992) and Dundes and Falassi (1975).

St Felix – hamlet, population 335, in the German-speaking Italian province of South Tyrol. Studied by Cole and Wolfe (1974).

Stilo – agrotown in Calabria left by the Tassoni family in 1933 (Pitkin, 1985).

Surughu – village studied by Weingrod (1968).

Syracuse – real name of city in Sicily where Mingione (1985) studied the impact of a petro-chemical plant.

Terrone – small agricultural village in Basilicata studied by Miller and Miller (1978).

Torregreca – southern Italian agrotown studied by Cornelison (1976).

Trasacco – agrotown in the Abruzzi studied by White (1980).

Tret – Italian Alpine village – population 238 – on the Romance side of the frontier between the South Tyrol province of Italy and the Trentino province. South Tyrol is German-speaking. In Tret a dialect of Romance, Nones, is spoken. Studied by Cole and Wolfe (1974).

Valmonte – community near Rome where the Tassoni family, studied by Pitkin (1985), have lived since 1933.

Villamaura – an agrotown in Sicily, Italy, studied by Jane and Peter Schneider (1976).

MALTA

Hal-Farrug – a village in Malta studied by Boissevain (1969) in 1960. Population 1,400.

Hass-Sajjied – a Maltese village studied by Koster (1984).

Kirkop – parish discussed by Boissevain (1984).

Kortin – town of 5,000 studied by Boissevain (1965).

Mellieha – village with a band discussed by Boissevain (1984).

Naxxar – village where Boissevain (1984) filmed Holy Week celebrations.

Qrendi – village discussed by Boissevain (1984).

Zurrieq – village discussed by Boissevain (1984).

MOROCCO

Meknes – real name of Moroccan city where Crapanzano (1973, 1980) studied the Hamadsha and the life history of Tuhami.

Ouled Filali – village in Morocco near the city of Taroudannt, studied by Dwyer (1982).

Sale – a Moroccan city studied by Brown (1976).

Sefrov – real name of Moroccan city where Rabinow (1977) worked.

Sidi Lahcem – village where Rabinow (1977) did his Moroccan fieldwork.

Taroudannt – Moroccan city in the Souss plain studied by Dwyer (1978).

THE NETHERLANDS

Elschberg – a village in Brabant, The Netherlands, studied by Bax (1987).

Muusland – village of 750 people where dairy farming was in decline when studied by Verrips (1975).

Roersel – a rural town in Brabant, The Netherlands, studied by Bax (1985a).

Utrecht – real city studied by Brunt (1989).

Yerseke – fishing town in The Netherlands studied by van Ginkel (1991).

PORTUGAL

Alto – village in the Monchique mountains in southern Portugal, studied by Jenkins (1979).

Alvoco das Varzeas – village of 640 people near Coimbra in central/northern Portugal, studied by Goldey (1983a).

Fatima – real name of major pilgrimage site in Portugal. The Virgin appeared there in 1917, and there are both Catholic and Russian Orthodox devotees.

Fontelas – hamlet in northern Portugal studied by O'Neill (1987).

Lama – one of three villages studied by the late Anthony Leeds (1987) in northern Portugal.

Lanheses – a parish along the Lima River in the Portugese district of Viana do Castelo, studied by Brettel (1985).

Nazare – fishing community in central Portugal studied by Brogger (1990) and previously by Mendonsa (1982).

Oliveria da Hospital – country town of 9,500 studied by Goldey (1983a).

Pova da Praia – fishing village on the south-east coast of Portugal (the Algarve) near the Spanish border with 763 inhabitants, studied by Johnson (1979).

Santo Vitoria – village in the south of Portugal studied by Leeds (1987).

São João das Lampas – parish of 363 people near Lisbon, Portugal, studied by Riegelhaupt (1967).

São Martinho – village inland from Opporto studied by Leeds (1987).

São Miguel – a rural parish in central Portugal studied by Riegelhaupt (1976).

Vila Branca – small town of 600 people in southern Portugal studied by Lawrence (1982).

Vila Cha – fishing village on the north coast of Portugal studied by Cole (1991).

Vila Velha – village in southern Portugal on the Spanish border studied by Cutileiro (1971).

SPAIN

Alcala de la Sierra – village in the mountains of Andalusia studied by Pitt-Rivers (1954).

Alcudia de Guadix – town in Granada area of Andalusia, Spain where the novel *The Three-Cornered Hat* was set. Research conducted by Rhoades (1979a).

Almonaster – a small town in Huelva province, south-west Spain – studied by Aguilera (1978).

Alto Panades – a juridical district in Catalonia, studied by Hansen (1977). In the 1970s it had a population of 45,000 in twenty-three villages and two towns.

Barcelona – real name of the capital of Catalonia, Spain. Studied by McDonogh (1986a), Woolard (1989) and Hansen (1977).

Becedas – in Old Castile, Spain, studied by Brandes (1975). Population of 805 in 1970.

Belmonte de los Caballeros – in Aragon, studied by Lison-Tolosana (1966).

Belunya – a village in northern Catalonia studied by Asano-Tamanoi (1987).

Benabarre – a village in the Huesca province of Spain (that is the province on the French border), studied by Barrett (1974).

Cambrils – tourist resort on the Costa Dorada studied by Hermans (1981).

Cap Lloc – fishing village in Catalonia, Spain (the Costa Brava), now a major tourist centre, studied by Pi-Sunyer (1989).

Echalar – village in the Basque region of Spain studied by Douglas (1975).

El Palmar – fishing and farming village on the lake of Albufera de Valencia studied by Sanmartin (1982).

Elgeta – a village in the Basque area of Spain studied by Heiberg (1989). Near Mondragon.

Escalona – a small Andalusian plains town studied by Uhl (1985).

Ezquioga – in the Basque region of Spain where two children saw the Virgin Mary in July 1931. Researched by Christian (1987). The Virgin spoke to them in Euskera (Basque).

Farol – remote Catalonian fishing village where travel writer Lewis (1984) lived and worked as a fisherman in the 1930s.

Formentera – real name of small island in the Balearic group off the coast of Spain studied by Bestard-Camps (1991).

Fuenmayor – agrotown in the Guadalquivir River basin in Andalusia, studied by Gilmore (1980). Population 8,000.

Fuenterrabia – real name of town in the Basque country with a *parador* and a folk celebration, the *alarde*, studied by Greenwood (1976).

Granada – real name of Andalusian city studied by Slater (1990).

Grazalema – the real name of Alcala (see above).

Hogar – village of 825 people on the south face of the Pyrenees, studied by Adams (1971).

Ibiecca – village in Aragon, Spain, studied by Harding (1984).

Lluc – real name of pilgrimage site in Mallorca, the largest Balearic island of Spain. There is a statue of a (black) madonna housed in a large chapel.

Los Santos – village on Tenerife, Canary Islands, studied by Moore (1976b).

Melilla – a Spanish enclave in Morocco. A small port held by Spain since the 1490s. Studied by Driessen (1992).

Mirabuenos – a small town near Cordoba in Andalusia, Spain, studied by Driessen (1984).

Monteros – agrotown in Andalusia studied by Brandes (1980).

Murelaga – village in the Basque region of Spain studied by Douglass (1969).

Nansa Valley – area in northern Spain, near Santander, where Christian (1972) worked.

Navanogal – settlement of 800 people west of Madrid studied by Brandes (1975).

Palma – capital city of Spanish Balearic island of Mallorca. Work-place of the Xueta studied by Moore (1976a).

Ramosierra – in Soria, Old Castile north-east of Madrid, with a population of 1,460 in 1954, studied by Kenny (1960).

Ronda – real name of town in Andalusia with population of 30,000 in 1979. Studied over twenty years by John and Marie Corbin (1983, 1987).

Saburneda – capital of the Valle de Solan, a village in the central Pyrenees studied by Codd (1971) (later Redclift) with a hydro-electric scheme and a population of 1,260.

Santa Maria – village between La Coruna and Santiago de Compostella in Galicia studied by Buechler (1987).

Santa Maria de Monte – a village in Leon with 120 permanent residents in 1980, studied by Behar (1986).

Seville – city in Andalusia, Spain, with 600,000 inhabitants in 1979. Base for research by Press (1979).

Tajos – village in the hills behind Malaga, where life histories were collected by Fraser (1973).

Tudanca – village in the Nansa Valley (see above).

Vado de las Chozas – village in Andalusia with about 3,000 inhabitants, studied by Guarino (1991).

Valdemora del Castillo – hamlet with eleven families in Old Castile, Spain, studied by Freeman (1973).

SWITZERLAND

Bagnes – a mountain commune in Switzerland studied by Weinberg (1975).

Bruson – one of the ten villages in the commune of Bagnes (see above).

Kippel – Alpine village researched by John Friedl (1974).

Thoune – destination for Galician guestworkers studied by Buechler (1987).

Torbel – Alpine village studied by Netting (1981).

Vernamiege – Alpine village studied by Berthoud (1967).

TURKEY

Ziyaret – town studied by Nancy Tapper (1990).

UK AND THE REPUBLIC OF IRELAND

Ashton – Yorkshire mining village studied by Dennis *et al.* (1957).

Ballybran – village in west Ireland studied by Scheper-Hughes (1979).

Blaenau Ffestiniog – real name of a small industrial town in North Wales, studied by Emmett (1982a).

Clachan – three townships in Lewis, near the capital of the island, Stornoway, studied by Mewett (1982).

Elmdon – real name of Essex village near Cambridge where anthropologists did a community study in the 1960s (see Strathern, 1981).

Geall – a Gaelic-speaking, crofting community on the island of Lewis, in the Outer Hebrides, Scotland, studied by Parman (1990).

Gislea – village in the fenlands studied by Chamberlain (1975).

Gosforth – village in Cumbria, north-west England, studied by Williams (1956).

Hull – real name of city and port in north-west England where fishing fleets were studied by Tunstall (1972).

Kilbroney – a small village in Northern Ireland, on the coast south of Belfast. Population 4,000. Studied by Larsen (1982a, b).

Knock – real name of pilgrimage site in County Mayo, Republic of Ireland.

Llan – north Wales village studied by Emmett (1964).

Llanfighangel yng Ngwynfa – Welsh villiage studied by Rees (1950).

Llanfrothen – real name of Llan (see above).

Petrediwaith – village on the Welsh border studied by Frankenberg (1957).

Tory Island – island 9 miles off the coast of Donegal, Ireland, with 300 Gaelic-speaking Roman Catholics. Studied by Fox (1978).

Westrigg – village in the Cheviots, on the Scottish border, studied by Littlejohn (1964).

Whalsay – an 8-mile-square island community off the coast of the main Shetland Island, studied by Cohen (1982).

YUGOSLAVIA

Medjugorje – real name of town in Hercegovina, Yugoslavia, where the Virgin Mary appeared in 1981. Studied by Bax (1992).

References

Abeles, M. (1991) *Quiet Days in Burgundy*, Cambridge: Cambridge University Press.

Aceves, J.B. and Douglass, W. (eds) (1976) *The Changing Faces of Rural Spain*, New York: Wiley.

Adams, P. (1971) Public and private interests in Hogar. In F.G. Bailey (ed.) *Gifts and Poison*, Oxford: Basil Blackwell.

Aggleton, P., Homans, H. and Warwick, I. (1988) Young people's health beliefs about AIDS. In P. Aggleton and H. Homans (eds) *Social Aspects of AIDS*, London: Falmer.

Aggleton, P., Homans, H. and Warwick, I. (1989) Health education, sexuality and AIDS. In S. Walker and L. Barton (eds) *Politics and the Process of Schooling*, Milton Keynes: Open University Press.

Aguilera, F.E. (1978) *St Eulalia's People*, St Paul, MN: West Publishing Co.

Allum, P.A. (1973) *Politics and Society in Post-War Naples*, Cambridge: Cambridge University Press.

Amin, A.(1985) Restructuring in Fiat and the decentralisation of production into Southern Italy. In R. Hudson and J. Lewis (eds) *Uneven Development in Southern Europe*, London: Methuen.

Anderson, R.T. and Anderson, B.G. (1962) Replicate social structure, *Southwestern Journal of Anthropology* 18, 365–370.

Anderson, R.T. and Anderson, B.G. (1964) *The Vanishing Village*, Seattle, WA: University of Washington Press.

Appel, Willa (1976) The myth of the *jettatura*. In C. Maloney (ed.) *The Evil Eye*, New York: Columbia University Press.

Ardener, E. (1972) Belief and the problem of women. In J. Lafontaine (ed.) *The Interpretation of Ritual*, London: Tavistock.

Ardener, E. (1975) The 'problem' revisited. In S. Ardener (ed.) *Perceiving Women*, London: Dent.

Ardener, S. (ed.) (1975) *Perceiving Women*, London: Dent.

Ardener, S. (ed.) (1978) *Defining Female*, London: Croom Helm.

Ardener, S. (ed.) (1981) *Women and Space*, London: Croom Helm.

Ardener, S. (1985) The social anthropology of women and feminist anthropology, *Anthropology Today* 1, 5, 24–26.

Arensberg, C. (1937) *The Irish Countryman*, New York: Macmillan.

Arensberg, C.M. and Kimball, S.T. (1940) *Family and Community in Ireland*, London: Peter Smith.

Asano-Tamanoi, M. (1987) Shame, family and state in Catalonia and Japan. In D. Gilmore (ed.) *Honour and Shame and the Unity of the Mediterranean*, Washington, DC: American Anthropological Association.

Aschenbrenner, S. (1986) *Life in a Changing Greek Village*, Dubuque, IA, Iowa: Kendall/Hunt.

Atkinson, P.A. (1990) *The Ethnographic Imagination*, London: Routledge.

Atkinson, P.A. (1992) *Understanding Ethnographic Texts*, London: Sage.

Badone, E. (1989) *The Appointed Hour*, Berkeley, CA: University of California Press.

Badone, E. (1990) Breton folklore of anticlericalism. In E. Badone (ed.) *Religious Orthodoxy and Popular Faith in European Society*, Princeton: Princeton University Press.

Bailey, F.G. (1971a) Gifts and poison. In F.G. Bailey (ed.) *Gifts and Poison*, Oxford: Basil Blackwell.

Bailey, F.G. (1971b) Changing communities. In F.G. Bailey (ed.) *Gifts and Poison*, Oxford: Basil Blackwell.

Bailey, F.G. (1971c) What are Signori? In F.G. Bailey (ed.) *Gifts and Poison*, Oxford: Basil Blackwell.

Banfield, E. (1958) *The Moral Basis of a Backward Society*, New York: Free Press.

Barrett, R.A. (1974) *Benabarre*, New York: Holt, Rinehart and Winston. (2nd edn, 1986, Prospect Heights, IL: Waveland Press.)

Bastenier, A. and Dassetto, F. (1988) Work and the indeterminate status of young North Africans and Turks in Belgium. In C. Wilpert (ed.) *Entering the Working World*, Aldershot: Gower.

Bax, Mart (1983a) 'Us' Catholics and 'Them' Catholics in Dutch Brabant, *Anthropological Quarterly* 56, 167–178.

Bax, Mart (1985a) Religious infighting and the formation of a dominant Catholic regime in southern Dutch society, *Social Compass* 32, 1, 57–72.

Bax, Mart (1985b) Popular devotions, power and religious regimes in Catholic Dutch Brabant, *Ethnology* 24, 215–227.

Bax, Mart (1987) Religious regimes and state formation, *Anthropological Quarterly* 60, 1–12.

Bax, Mart (1988) Return to mission status? *Ethnologia Europaea* 18, 73–79.

Bax, Mart (1991) Marian apparitions in Medjugorge. In E. Wolf (ed.) *Religious Regimes and State Formation*, Albany, NY: SUNY Press.

Bax, Mart (1992) Women's madness in Medjugorje, *Journal of Mediterranean Studies* 2, 1, 41–53.

Behar, R. (1986) *Santa Maria del Monte*, Princeton, NJ: Princeton University Press.

Bell, C. and Newby, H. (1971) *Community Studies*, London: Allen & Unwin.

Belmonte, T. (1979) *The Broken Fountain*, New York: Columbia University Press.

Belmonte, T. (1983) Social life in subproletarian Naples. In M. Kenny and D. Kertzer (eds) *Urban Life in Mediterranean Europe*, Urbana, IL: University of Illinois Press.

Belmonte, T. (1989) *The Broken Fountain* (2nd edition), New York: Columbia University Press.

Berger, A.H. (1986) *Cooperation, Conflict, and Production Environment in Highland Sardinia.* Ann Arbor, MI: UMI Press.

Berkowitz, Susan G. (1984) Familism, kinship and sex roles, *Anthropological Quarterly* 57, 2, 83–92.

Bernard, H.R. and Ashton-Vouyoucalos, S. (1976) Return migration to Greece, *Journal of the Stewart Anthropological Society* 8, 1, 31–35.

Berthoud, G. (1967) *Changements Economiques et Sociaux de la Montagne,* Berne: Editions Francke.

Bestard-Camps, Joan (1991) *What's in a Relative?* Oxford: Berg.

Blaxter, L. (1971) *Rendre service,* and *Jalousie.* In F.G. Bailey (ed.) *Gifts and Poison,* Oxford: Basil Blackwell.

Blok, A. (1974) *The Mafia of a Sicilian Village 1860–1960,* New York: Harper & Row.

Boatswain, T. and Nicolson, C. (1989) *A Traveller's History of Greece,* Moreton-in-Marsh: Windrush Press.

Boissevain, J. (1965) *Saints and Fireworks,* London: Athlone.

Boissevain, J. (1969) *Hal-Farrug: A Village in Malta,* New York: Holt, Rinehart & Winston.

Boissevain, J. (1974) *Friends of Friends,* Oxford: Basil Blackwell.

Boissevain, J. (1975) Introduction: Towards a social anthropology of Europe. In J. Boissevain and E. Friedl (eds) *Beyond the Community,* The Hague: University of Amsterdam.

Boissevain, J. (1977) When the saints go marching out. In E. Gellner and J. Waterbury (eds) *Patrons and Clients in Mediterranean Societies,* London: Duckworth.

Boissevain, J. (1979) Notes towards a social anthropology of the Mediterranean, *Current Anthropology* 20, 81–93.

Boissevain, J. (1980) *Hal-Farrug: A Village in Malta* (2nd edition), New York: Holt, Rinehart & Winston.

Boissevain, J. (1984) Ritual escalation in Malta. In E.R. Wolf (ed.) *Religion, Power and Protest in Local Communities,* Berlin: Mouton.

Boissevain, J. (n.d.) Lecture delivered at the University of Malta.

Boisvert, C.C. (1987) Working-class Portuguese families in a French provincial town. In H.C. Buechler and J.M. Buechler (eds) *Migrants in Europe,* New York: Greenwood Press.

Bott, E. (1971) *Family and Social Networks,* London: Routledge.

Bourdieu, P. (1971) The Berber house. In M. Douglas (ed.) *Rules and Meanings,* Harmondsworth: Penguin.

Brandes, S. (1975) *Migration, Kinship and Community,* New York: Academic Press.

Brandes, S. (1980) *Metaphors of Masculinity,* Philadelphia, PA: University of Pennsylvania Press.

Brandes, S. (1981) Like wounded stags. In S. Ortner and H. Whitehead (eds) *Sexual Meanings,* Cambridge: Cambridge University Press.

Brandes, S. (1985) Women of southern Spain. In D. Gilmore and G. Gwynne (eds) *Sex and Gender in Southern Europe.* A Special Issue of *Anthropology* 9, 1 and 2, 111–128.

Brandes, S. (1987) Reflections on honour and shame in the Mediterranean. In D. Gilmore (ed.) *Honour and Shame and the Unity of the Mediterranean*, Washington, DC: American Anthropological Association.

Brandes, S. (1992) Sex roles and anthropological research in rural Andalusia. In J. de Pina-Cabral and J. Campbell (eds) *Europe Observed*, London: Macmillan.

Brettell, C.B. (1985) Male migrants and unwed mothers. In D. Gilmore and G. Gwynne (eds) *Sex and Gender in Southern Europe*. A Special Issue of *Anthropology* 9, 1 and 2, 87–110.

Brettell, C. (1986) *Men who Migrate, Women who Wait*, Princeton, NJ: Princeton University Press.

Brogger, J. (1971) *Montevarese*, Oslo: Universitetsforlaget.

Brogger, J. (1990) *Pre-Bureaucratic Europeans*, Oslo: Norwegian University Press.

Brown, K. (1976) *People of Sale*, Manchester: Manchester University Press.

Brunt, L. (1989) Foreigners in the neighbourhood. In J. Boissevain and J. Verrips (eds) *Dutch Dilemmas*, Maastricht: West Germany.

Buechler, H. (1983) Spanish urbanization from a grassroots perspective. In M. Kenny and D. Kertzer (eds) *Urban Life in Mediterranean Europe*, Urbana, IL: University of Illinois Press.

Buechler, H. (1987) Spanish Galician migration to Switzerland. In H.C. Buechler and J.M. Buechler (eds) *Migrants in Europe*, New York: Greenwood Press.

Buechler, H. and Buechler, J.M. (1981) *Carmen*, Cambridge, MA.: Schenkman.

Buechler, H.C. and Buechler, J.M. (eds) (1987) *Migrants in Europe*, New York: Greenwood Press.

Burawoy, Michael (ed.) (1991) *Ethnography Unbound*, Berkeley: University of California Press.

Burgnière, A. (1977) *Bretons de Plozevet*, Paris: Flammorion.

Burman, S. (ed.) (1979) *Fit Work for Women*, London: Croom Helm.

Calabresi, Ann T. (1987) Vin Santo and wine in a Tuscan farmhouse. In M. Douglas (ed.) *Constructive Drinking*, Cambridge: Cambridge University Press.

Callan, H. and Ardener, S. (eds) (1984) *The Incorporated Wife*, London: Croom Helm.

Camilleri, C. (1986) *Cultural Anthropology and Education*, London: Kogan Page.

Campbell, J.K. (1964) *Honour, Family and Patronage*, Oxford: Clarendon Press.

Campbell, J.K. (1992) Fieldwork among the Sarakatsani 1954–1955. In J. de Pina-Cabral and J. Campbell (eds) *Europe Observed*, London: Macmillan.

Caraveli, A. (1980) Bridge between worlds, *Journal of American Folklore* 93, 129–157.

Caraveli, A. (1982) The song beyond the song, *Journal of American Folklore* 95, 129–58.

Caraveli, A. (1985) The symbolic village, *Journal of American Folklore* 98, 259–86.

Catedra, Maria (1992) *This World, Other Worlds*, Chicago, IL: University of Chicago Press.

Chamberlain, M. (1975) *Fenwomen*, London: Virago.

Chapman, C. Gower (1971) *Milocca*, Cambridge, MA: Schenkman.

Chapman, M. (1978) *The Gaelic Vision in Scottish Culture*, London: Croom Helm.

Chapman, M. (1992) Fieldwork, language, and locality in Europe, from the North. In J. de Pina-Cabral and J. Campbell (eds) *Europe Observed*, London: Macmillan.

Charsley, S.R. (1991) *Rites of Marrying*, Manchester: Manchester University Press.

Christian, W.A. (1972) *Person and God in a Spanish Valley*, New York: Seminar Press. (2nd edn, 1989, Princeton, NJ: Princeton University Press.)

Christian, W.A. (1987) Tapping and defining new power, *American Ethnologist* 14, 1, 140–166.

Christian, W.A. (1991) Secular and religious responses to a child's potentially fatal illness. In E.R. Wolf (ed.) *Religious Regimes and State Formation*. Albany, NY: SUNY Press.

Chubb, J. (1982) *Patronage, Power and Poverty in Southern Italy*, Cambridge: Cambridge University Press.

Clout, H. (1984) *A Rural Policy for the EEC?* London: Methuen.

Codd, N. (1971) Reputation and social structure in a Spanish Pyrenean village. In F.G. Bailey (ed.) *Gifts and Poison*, Oxford: Basil Blackwell.

Cohen, A.P. (ed.) (1982) *Belonging*, Manchester: Manchester University Press.

Colclough, N.T. (1971) Social mobility and social control in a Southern Italian village. In F.G. Bailey (ed.) *Gifts and Poison*, Oxford: Basil Blackwell.

Cole, J.W. (1977) Anthropology comes part-way home, *Annual Review of Anthropology* 6, 349–378.

Cole, J.W. and Wolf, E.R. (1974) *The Hidden Frontier*, New York: Academic Press.

Cole, S. (1991) *Women of the Praia*, Princeton: Princeton University Press.

Connell, C. (1980) *In the Bee-loud Glade*, Napflion: Peloponnesian Folklore Foundation.

Corbin, J. (1979) Social class and patron-clientage in Andalusia, *Anthropological Quarterly* 52, 2, 99–114.

Corbin, J. and Corbin, M. (1983) *Compromising Relations*, Farnborough: Gower.

Corbin, J. and Corbin, M. (1987) *Urbane Thought*, Farnborough: Gower.

Cornelisen, A. (1976) *Women of the Shadows*, New York: Vintage.

Cornelisen, A. (1980) *Flight from Torregreca*, London: Macmillan.

Counihan, C.M. (1985) Transvestism and gender in a Sardinian carnival. In D. Gilmore and G. Gwynne (eds) *Sex and Gender in Southern Europe*. A Special Issue of *Anthropology* 9, 1 and 2, 11–24.

Cowan, Jane K. (1990) *Dance and the Body Politic in Northern Greece*, Princeton, NJ: Princeton University Press.

Cowan, Jane K. (1991) Going out for coffee? In P. Loizos and E. Papataxiarchis (eds) *Contested Identities*, Princeton, NJ: Princeton University Press.

Crapanzano, V. (1973) *The Hamadsha*, Berkeley, CA: University of California Press.

Crapanzano, V. (1980) *Tuhami*, Chicago, IL: University of Chicago Press.

Crapanzano, V. (1985) *Waiting*, London: Granada.

Crewe, Q. (1980) *International Pocket Food Book*, London: Mitchell Beazley.

Cronin, C. (1970) *The Sting of Change*, Chicago: University of Chicago Press.

Cross, M. (1988) Ethnic minority youth in a collapsing labour market. In C. Wilpert (ed.) *Entering the Working World*, Aldershot: Gower.

Crump, T. (1975) The context of European anthropology. In J. Boissevain and E. Friedl (eds) *Beyond the Community*, The Hague: University of Amsterdam.

Cucchiari, Salvatore (1988) Adapted for heaven, *American Ethnologist* 15, 417–441.

Cutileiro, J. (1971) *A Portuguese Rural Society*, Oxford: Clarendon Press.

Dahlberg, A. (1991) The body as a principle of holism. In J. Eade and M. Sallnow (eds) *Contesting the Sacred*, London: Routledge.

Danforth, L. (1982) *The Death Rituals of Rural Greece*, Princeton, NJ: Princeton University Press.

Danforth, L. (1989) *Fire Walking and Religious Healing*, Princeton, NJ: Princeton University Press.

Darmanin, M. (1990) Unpublished PhD Thesis, University of Wales, Cardiff.

David, E. (1955) *Mediterranean Food*, Harmondsworth: Penguin.

David, E. (1964) *French Provincial Cooking*, Harmondsworth: Penguin.

Davis, J. (1970) Morals and backwardness, *Comparative Studies in Society and History* 12, 3: 340–353.

Davis, J. (1973) *Land and Family in a South Italian Town*, London: Athlone Press.

Davis, J. (1977) *People of the Mediterranean*, London: Routledge.

Day, G. and Rees, G. (eds) (1991) *Regions, Nations and European Integration*, Cardiff: University of Wales Press.

Delamont, S. (1983) Salmon, chicken, cake and tears. In A. Murcott (eds) *The Sociology of Food and Eating*, Farnborough: Gower.

Delamont, S. (1987) S4C and the grassroots, *Contemporary Wales* 1, 53–72.

Delamont, S. (1989) *Knowledegable Women*, London: Routledge.

Delamont, S. (1991) The HIT LIST and other horror stories, *The Sociological Review* 39, 2, 238–259.

Delamont, S. and Duffin, L. (eds) (1978) *The Nineteenth Century Woman*, London: Croom Helm.

Dennis, N., Henriques, F. and Slaughter, C. (1957) *Coal is our Life*, London: Routledge & Kegan Paul.

Di Giacomo, S.M. (1987) 'La Caseta i l'Hortet', rural imagery in Catalan urban politics, *Anthropological Quarterly* 60, 4 160–166.

Dionisopoulis-Mass, R. (1976) Nisi. In M. Dimen and E. Friedl (eds)

Regional Variation in Modern Greece and Cyprus, New York: Annals of the New York Academy of Sciences.

Douglas, M. (ed.) (1975) *Implicit Meanings*, London: Routledge.

Douglas, M.(ed.) (1987) *Constructive Drinking*, Cambridge: Cambridge University Press.

Douglass, W.A. (1969) *Death in Murelaga*, Seattle, WA: University of Washington Press.

Douglass, W.A. (1975) *Echalar and Murelaga*, New York: St Martin's Press.

Douglass, W.A. (1980) The south Italian family, *Journal of Family History* 5, 338–359.

Douglass, W.A. (1983) Migration in Italy. In M. Kenny and D. Kertzer (eds) *Urban Life in Mediterranean Europe*, Urbana, IL: University of Illinois Press.

Douglass, W.A. (1984) *Emigration in a South Italian Town*, New Brunswick, NJ: Rutgers University Press.

Driessen, H. (1983) Male sociability and rituals of masculinity in rural Andalusia, *Anthropological Quarterly* 56, 3, 125–131.

Driessen, H. (1984) Religious brotherhoods. In E. Wolf (ed.) *Religion, Power and Protest in Local Communities*, Berlin: Mouton.

Driessen, H. (1992) *On the Spanish–Moroccan Frontier*, Oxford: Berg.

Dubisch, J. (1986) Culture enters through the kitchen. In J. Dubisch (ed.) *Gender and Power in Rural Greece*, Princeton, NJ: Princeton University Press.

Dubisch, J. (1988) Golden oranges and silver ships, *Journal of Modern Greek Studies* 6, 117–134.

Dubisch, J. (1990) Pilgrimage and popular religion at a Greek holy shrine. In E. Badone (ed.) *Religious Orthodoxy and Popular Faith in European Society*, Princeton, NJ: Princeton University Press.

Dubisch, J. (1991) Gender, kinship and religion. In P. Loizos and E. Papataxiarchis (eds) *Contested Identities*, Princeton, NJ: Princeton University Press.

du Boulay, J. (1974) *Portrait of a Greek Mountain Village*, Oxford: Clarendon Press.

du Boulay, J. (1982) The Greek vampire, *Man* 17, 219–238.

du Boulay, J. (1991) Strangers and gifts, *Journal of Mediterranean Studies* 1, 1, 37–53.

Dundes, A. and Falassi, A. (1975) *La terra in piazza*, Berkeley, CA: University of California Press.

Dwyer, Daisy H. (1978) *Images and Self-Images*, New York: Columbia University Press.

Dwyer, Kevin (1982) *Moroccan Dialogues*, Baltimore, MD: Johns Hopkins University Press.

Eade, J. (1991) Order and power at Lourdes. In J. Eade and M. Sallnow (eds) *Contesting the Sacred*, London: Routledge.

Eickelman, D. (1976) *Moroccan Islam*, Austin, TX: University of Texas Press.

Eickelman, D. (1981) *The Middle East*, Englewood Cliffs, NJ: Prentice Hall.

Eickelman, D. (1985) *Knowledge and Power in Morocco*, Princeton, NJ: Princeton University Press.

Eldering, L. and Kloprogge, J. (eds) (1989) *Different Cultures, Same School*, Amsterdam: Swets & Zeitlinger.

Elyan, O. *et al.* (1978) RP-accented female speech. In P. Trudgill (ed.) *Sociolinguistic Patterns in British English*, London: Edward Arnold.

Emmett, I. (1964) *A North Wales Parish*, London: Routledge.

Emmett, I. (1982a) *Fe godwn ni eto.* In A Cohen (ed.) *Belonging*, Manchester: Manchester University Press.

Emmett, I. (1982b) Place, community and bilingualism in Blaenau Festiniog. In A. Cohen (ed.) *Belonging*, Manchester: Manchester University Press.

Evans, J. (1982) 'Anti-Welsh influences'. Letter published in *The Western Mail*, December 23rd, p. 10.

Evans, N. (1991) Internal colonialism? In G. Day and G. Rees (eds) *Regions, Nations and European Integration*, Cardiff: University of Wales Press.

Favret-Saada, J. (1980) *Deadly Words*, Cambridge: Cambridge University Press.

Favret-Saada, J. (1989) Unwitching as therapy, *American Ethnologist* 16, 1, 40–56.

Fermor, P.L. (1958) *Mani*, London: John Murray.

Fermor, P.L. (1966) *Roumeli*, London: John Murray.

Fernandez, J.W. (1983) Consciousness and class in Southern Spain, *American Ethnologist* 10, 165–173.

Fernandez, J.W. (1987) Fieldwork in southwestern Europe, *Critique of Anthropology* 7, 1, 83–85.

Fibbi, R. and Rham, G. (1988) Switzerland. In C. Wilpert (ed.) *Entering the Working World*, Aldershot: Gower.

Filippucci, P. (1992) Tradition in action: the *carnevale* of Bascano, 1824–1989, *Journal of Mediterranean Studies* 2, 55–68.

Flecker, J.E. (1947) *Collected Poems*, London: Secker & Warburg.

Fox, R. (1978) *The Tory Islanders*, Cambridge: Cambridge University Press.

Frankenberg, R. (1957) *Village on the Border*, London: Cohen & West.

Frankenberg, R. (1966) *Communities in Britain*, Harmondsworth: Penguin.

Franklin, S.H. (1969) *The European Peasantry*, London: Methuen.

Fraser, R. (1973) *The Pueblo*, London: Allen Lane.

Freeman, S.T. (1967) Religious aspects of the social organization of a Castilian village, *American Anthropologist* 70, 34–49.

Freeman, S.T. (1970) *Neighbours*, Chicago: University of Chicago Press.

Freeman, S.T. (1973) Studies in rural European social organization, *American Anthropologist* 75, 743–750.

Freeman, S.T. (1979) *The Pasiegos*, Chicago: University of Chicago Press.

Friedl, E. (1962) *Vasilika: A Village in Modern Greece*, New York: Holt, Rinehart & Winston.

Friedl, J. (1974) *Kippel*, New York: Holt, Rinehart & Winston.

Gaines, Atwood D. (1985) Faith, fashion and family, *Anthropological Quarterly* 58, 47–62.

Galt, A.H. (1974) Rethinking patron–client relationships, *Anthropological Quarterly* 47, 182–202.

Galt, A.H. (1982) The evil eye as synthetic image and its meaning on the island of Pantellaria, Italy, *American Ethnologist* 9, 664–682.

Galt, A.H. (1984/5) Does the Mediterraneanist dilemma have straw horns? *American Ethnologist* 12, 2, 369–371.

Galt, A.H. (1991) *Far from the Church Bells: Settlement and Society in an Apulian Town*, Cambridge: Cambridge University Press.

Gerholm, T. and Lithman, Y.G. (eds) (1988) *The New Islamic Presence in Western Europe*, London: Mansell.

Giles, Wenona (1991) Class, gender and race struggles in a Portuguese neighbourhood in London, *International Journal of Urban and Regional Research* 15, 3, 432–441.

Gili, E. (1963) *Tia Victoria's Spanish Kitchen*, London: Nicholas Kaye.

Gilmore, D. (1980) *People of the Plain*, New York: Columbia University Press.

Gilmore, D. (1985) Review of J. and M. Corbin (1984) *Compromising Relations* in *Man* 20, 360–361.

Gilmore, D. (1987a) Honour, honesty and shame. In D. Gilmore (ed.) *Honour and Shame and the Unity of the Mediterranean*, Washington, DC: American Anthropological Association.

Gilmore, D. (1987b) Introduction: The shame of dishonour. In D. Gilmore (ed.) *Honour and Shame and the Unity of the Mediterranean*, Washington, DC: American Anthropological Association.

Gilmore, D. (1990) On Mediterraneanist studies, *Current Anthropology* 31, 395–396.

Gilmore, D. and Gwynne, G. (eds) (1985) *Sex and Gender in Southern Europe*. A special Issue of *Anthropology* 9, 1 and 2.

Gilsenan, M. (1982) *Recognising Islam*, London: Croom Helm.

Ginzburg, C. (1980) *The Cheese and the Worms*, London: Routledge.

Ginzburg, C. (1983) *The Night Battles*, London: Routledge.

Giovannini, M.J. (1986) Female anthropologist and male informant. In T.L. Whitehead and M.E. Conaway (eds) *Self, Sex and Gender in Cross-Cultural Fieldwork*, Urbana, IL: University of Illinois Press.

Glaser, B. and Strauss, A.L. (1965) *Time for Dying*, Chicago, IL: Aldine.

Golde, G. (1975) *Catholics and Protestants*, New York: Academic Press.

Goldey, P. (1983a) Migration, cooperation and development In R. Kubat (ed.) *The Politics of Return*, New York: Centre for Migration Studies.

Goldey, P. (1983b) The good death. In P. Feijo, H. Martins and J. Pina-Cabral (eds) *Death in Portugal*, Oxford: Department of Social Anthropology.

Goodman, C. (1987) A day in the life of a single Spanish woman in West Germany. In H.C. Buechler and J.M. Buechler (eds) *Migrants in Europe*, New York: Greenwood Press.

Graburn, Nelson H.H. (1989) Tourism: the sacred journey. In V. Smith (ed.) *Hosts and Guests* (2nd edition), Philadelphia, PA: University of Pennsylvania Press.

Graddol, D. and Swann, J. (1989) *Gender Voices*, Oxford: Blackwell.

Greenwood, D.J. (1976) *Unrewarding Wealth*, Cambridge: Cambridge University Press.

Greenwood, D.J. (1989) Culture by the pound. In V.L. Smith (ed.) *Hosts and Guests* (2nd edition), Philadelphia: University of Pennsylvania Press.

Gregory, D.D. (1976) Migration and demographic change in Andalusia. In J.B. Aceves and W. Douglass (eds) *The Changing Faces of Rural Spain*, New York: Wiley.

Gregory, D.D. and Cazorla Perez, J. (1985) Intra-European migration and regional development. In R. Rogers (ed.) *Guests Come to Stay*, Boulder, CO: Westview Press.

Grigson, J. (1983) *The Observer Guide to European Cookery*, London: Michael Joseph.

Grillo, R.D. (1985) *Ideologies and Institutions in Urban France*, Cambridge: Cambridge University Press.

Grillo, R.D. (1989a) *Dominant Languages*, Cambridge: Cambridge University Press.

Grillo, R.D. (ed.) (1989b) *Social Anthropology and the Politics of Language*, London: Routledge.

Guarino, M. (1991) El Niño que no Llora no Marna: Patronage and protest in an Andalusian village, *Journal of Mediterranean Studies* 1, 68–86.

Gurr, Lisa A. (1987) Maigret's Paris, conserved and distilled. In M. Douglas (ed.) *Constructive Drinking*, Cambridge: Cambridge University Press.

Halpern, J.M. (1987) Yugoslav migration process and employment in western Europe. In H.C. Buechler and J.M. Buechler (eds) *Migrants in Europe*, New York: Greenwood Press.

Hammersley, M. and Atkinson, P. (1983) *Ethnography*, London: Routledge.

Hansen, E.C. (1977) *Rural Catalonia under the Franco Regime*, Cambridge: Cambridge University Press.

Hansen, E.C. (1987) Foreword, *Anthropological Quarterly* 60, 4, 150–151.

Harding, S. (1984) *Remaking Ibieca: Agrarian Reform in Aragon under Franco*, Chapel Hill, NC: University of North Carolina Press.

Heaton, V. (1975) *Wedding Etiquette Properly Explained* (4th edition), Kingswood, Surrey: Paperfronts.

Hechter, M. (1975) *Internal Colonialism*, London: Routledge.

Heiberg, M. (1989) *The Making of the Basque Nation*, Cambridge: Cambridge University Press.

Helias, P.J. (1978) *The Horse of Pride*, New Haven, CT: Yale University Press.

Henson, H. (1974) *British Social Anthropologists and Language*, Oxford: Clarendon Press.

Heppenstall, M.A. (1971) Reputation, criticism and information in an Austrian village. In F.G. Bailey (ed.) *Gifts and Poison*, Oxford: Basil Blackwell.

Hermans, D. (1981) The encounter of agriculture and tourism: a Catalan case, *Annals of Tourism Research* 8, 3, 462–479.

Hertz, R. (1913/1983) St Besse: a study of an Alpine cult. In S. Wilson (ed.) *Saints and their Cults*, Cambridge: Cambridge University Press.

Herzfeld, M. (1980) Honour and Shame, *Man* 15, 339–351.

Herzfeld, M. (1982) *Ours Once More*, Austin, TX: University of Texas Press.

Herzfeld, M. (1983) Semantic slippage and moral fall, *Journal of Modern Greek Studies* 1, 161–172.

Herzfeld, M. (1984) The horns of the Mediterraneanist dilemma, *American Ethnologist* 11, 439–454.

Herzfeld, M. (1985) *The Poetics of Manhood*, Princeton, NJ: Princeton University Press.

Herzfeld, M. (1987) *Anthropology through the Looking-glass*, Cambridge: Cambridge University Press.

Herzfeld, M. (1991) *A Place in History*, Princeton, NJ: Princeton University Press.

Hill, B. (1984) *The Common Agricultural Policy*, London: Methuen.

Hirschon, R.B. (1983) Under one roof. In M. Kenny and D. Kertzer (eds) *Urban Life in Mediterranean Europe*, Urbana, IL: University of Illinois Press.

Hirschon, R.B. (ed.) (1984) *Women and Property: Women as Property*, London: Croom Helm.

Hirschon, R.B. (1989) *Heirs of the Greek Catastrophe*, Oxford: Clarendon Press.

Hobsbawm, E.J. (1959) *Primitive Rebels*, Manchester: Manchester University Press.

Holden, P. (ed.) (1983) *Women's Religious Experience*, London: Croom Helm.

Holmes, D.R. (1983) A peasant–worker model in a northern Italian context, *American Ethnologist* 10, 734–748.

Holmes, D.R. (1989) *Cultural Disenchantments*, Princeton, NJ: Princeton University Press.

Hudson, R. (1992) Bizarre events in the old bazaar, *Times Higher Education Supplement*, 28 February: 12.

Hudson, R. and Lewis, J. (eds) (1985) *Uneven Development in Southern Europe*, London: Methuen.

Hutson, J. (1971) A politician in Valloire. In F.G. Bailey (ed.) *Gifts and Poison*, Oxford: Basil Blackwell.

Hutson, S. (1971) Social ranking in a French alpine community. In F.G. Bailey (ed.) *Debate and Compromise*, Oxford: Basil Blackwell.

Hutter, B. and Williams, G. (eds) (1981) *Controlling Women*, London: Croom Helm.

Jackson, A. (ed.) (1987) *Anthropology at Home*, London: Tavistock.

Jacobus, M. (ed.) (1979) *Women Writing and Writing about Women*, London: Croom Helm.

Jaffe, A. (1993) Involvement, detachment and representation on Corsica. In C.B. Brettell (ed.) *When They Read What We Write*, London: Bergin & Garvey.

Jenkins, R. (1979) *The Road to Alto*, London: Pluto.

Johnson, Twig (1979) Work together, eat together. In R. Anderson (ed.) *North Atlantic Maritime Cultures*, The Hague: Mouton/de Gruyter.

Jorion, Paul (1977) L'ordre moral dans une petite île de Bretagne, *Etudes rurales* 67, 31–45.

Jorion, P. (1982) The priest and the fisherman, *Man* 17, 275–86.

Just, R. (1991) The limits of kinship. In P. Loizos and E. Papataxiarchis (eds) *Contested Identities*, Princeton, NJ: Princeton University Press.

Kenna, M.E. (1976) Houses, fields and graves, *Ethnology* 15, 21–34.

Kenna, M.E. (1983) Institutional and transformational migration and the politics of community, *European Journal of Sociology* 24, 263–287.

Kenna, M.E. (1990) Family and economic life in a Greek island community. In C.C. Harris (ed.) *Family, Economy and Community*, Cardiff: University of Wales Press.

Kenna, M.E. (1991a) The power of the dead, *Journal of Mediterranean Studies* 1, 1, 101–119.

Kenna, M.E. (1991b) The social organization of exile, *Journal of Modern Greek Studies* 9, 1, 63–81.

Kenna, M.E. (1992) Changing places and altered perspectives. In J. Okely and H. Callaway (eds) *Anthropology and Autobiography*, London: Routledge.

Kenny, M. (1960) *A Spanish Tapestry*, London: Cohen & West.

Kenny, M. and Kertzer, D. (eds) (1983) *Urban Life in Mediterranean Europe*, Urbana, IL: University of Illinois Press.

Kenny, M. and Knipmeyer, M.C. (1983) Urban research in Spain. In M. Kenny and D. Kertzer (eds) *Urban Life in Mediterranean Europe*, Urbana, IL: University of Illinois Press.

Kertzer, D.I. (1980) *Comrades and Christians*, Cambridge: Cambridge University Press.

Kertzer, D.I. (1983) Urban research in Italy. In M. Kenny and D. Kertzer (eds) *Urban Life in Mediterranean Europe*, Urbana, IL: University of Illinois Press.

Kertzer, D.I. (1987) Childhood and industrialization in Italy, *Anthropological Quarterly* 60, 4, 152–159.

Kertzer, D.I. (1990) *Comrades and Christians* (2nd edition), Prospect Heights, IL: Waveland.

Kielstra, N. (1985) The rural Languedoc: periphery to 'relictual space'. In R. Hudson and J. Lewis (eds) *Uneven Development in Southern Europe*, London: Methuen.

King, R. (1979) Return migration, *Mediterranean Studies* 1, 2, 3–30.

King, R. (1984) Return migration and tertiary development, *Anthropological Quarterly* 53, 3, 112–124.

King, R. (ed.) (1986) *Return Migration and Regional Economic Problems*, London: Croom Helm.

King, R. (1987) *Italy*, London: Harper & Row.

King, R., Strachan, A. and Mortimer, J. (1986) Gastarbeiter go home. In R. King (ed.) *Return Migration and Regional Economic Problems*, London: Croom Helm.

Klinge, M. (1981) *A Brief History of Finland*, Helsinki: OTAVA.

Kofman, E. (1985) Dependent development in Corsica. In R. Hudson and J. Lewis (eds) *Uneven Development in Southern Europe*, London: Methuen.

Koster, A. (1984) The Kappillani. In E.R. Wolf (ed.) *Religion, Power and Protest in Local Communities*, Berlin: Mouton.

Ladurie, E. Le Roy (1975) *Montaillou*, London: Scola Press.

Larsen, S.S. (1982a) The two sides of the house. In A.P. Cohen (ed.) *Belonging*, Manchester: Manchester University Press.

Larsen, S.S. (1982b) The Glorious Twelfth. In A.P. Cohen (ed.) *Belonging*, Manchester: Manchester University Press.

Lawless, R. (1986) Return migration to Algeria. In R. King (ed.) *Return Migration and Regional Economic Problems*, London: Croom Helm.

Lawrence, D.L. (1982) Reconsidering the menstrual taboo, *Anthropological Quarterly* 55, 2, 84–98.

Layton, R. (1971) Patterns of informal interaction in Pellaport. In F.G. Bailey (ed.) *Gifts and Poison*, Oxford: Basil Blackwell.

Leach, E.R. (ed.) (1968) *The Dialectic in Practical Religion*, Cambridge: Cambridge University Press.

Leach, E.R. (1976) *Culture and Communication*, Cambridge: Cambridge University Press.

Leeds, A. (1987) Work, labour and their recompenses. In H.C. Buechler and J.M. Buechler (eds) *Migrants in Europe*, New York: Greenwood Press.

Leonard, D. (1980) *Sex and Generation*, London: Tavistock.

Levi, Carlo (1982) *Christ Stopped at Eboli*, Harmondsworth: Penguin.

Lewis, Norman (1984) *Voices of the Old Sea*, London: Hamish Hamilton.

Liebkind, K. (ed.) (1989) *New Identities in Europe*, Aldershot: Gower.

Linguistic Minorities Project (1985) *The Other Languages of England*, London: Routledge.

Lison-Tolosana, C. (1966) *Belmonte de los Caballeros*, London: Oxford University Press.

Lison-Tolosana, C. (1976) The ethics of inheritance. In J.G. Peristiany (ed.) *Mediterranean Family Structures*, Cambridge: Cambridge University Press.

Littlejohn, J. (1964) *Westrigg*, London: Routledge.

Llobera, J.R. (1986) Fieldwork in southwestern Europe, *Critique of Anthropology* 6, 2, 25–33.

Lodge, D. (1991) *Paradise News*, London: Secker & Warburg.

Loizos, P. (1975) *The Greek Gift*, Oxford: Basil Blackwell.

Loizos, P. (1981) *The Heart Grown Bitter*, Cambridge: Cambridge University Press.

Lopreato, J. (1967) *Peasants No More*, San Francisco, CA: Chandler Publishing Company.

Luhrmann, T. (1989) *Persuasions of the Witch's Craft*, Oxford: Basil Blackwell.

MacCannell, D. (1976) *The Tourist*, New York: Schocken.

McDonald, M. (1986) Celtic ethnic kinship and the problem of being English, *Current Anthropology* 27, 4, 333–341.

McDonald, M. (1987) The politics of fieldwork in Brittany. In A. Jackson (ed.) *Anthropology at Home*, London: Tavistock.

McDonald, M. (1989) *We are not French!* London: Routledge.

McDonald, M. (1993) The construction of difference. In S. McDonald (ed.) *Inside European Identities*, Oxford: Berg.

McDonald, Sharon (ed.) (1993) *Inside European Identities*, Oxford: Berg.

McDonogh, G.W. (1986a) *Good Families of Barcelona*, Princeton, NJ: Princeton University Press.

McDonogh, G.W. (ed.) (1986b) *Conflict in Catalonia*, Gainesville, FL: University of Florida Press.

McDonogh, G.W. (1987) The geography of evil, *Anthropological Quarterly* 60, 4, 174–184.

Machin, B. (1983) St George and the Virgin, *Social Analysis* 14, 107–126.

McKechnie, R. (1993) Becoming Celtic in Corsica. In S. McDonald (ed.) *Inside European Identities*, Oxford: Berg.

McKevitt, C. (1991a) To suffer and never to die, *Journal of Mediterranean Studies* 1, 1, 54–67.

McKevitt, C. (1991b) San Giovanni Rotondo and the shrine of Padre Pío. In J. Eade and M. Sallnow (eds) *Contesting the Sacred*, London: Routledge.

Mackinnon, K. (1987a) *Gender, Occupational and Educational Factors in Gaelic Language Regeneration*, Hatfield: Hatfield Polytechnic.

Makris, J. (1992) Ethnography, history, and collective representations. In J. de Pina-Cabral and J. Campbell (eds) *Europe Observed*, London: Macmillan.

Mandel, R. (1990) Shifting centres and emergent identities. In D.F. Eickelman and J. Piscatori (eds) *Muslim Travellers*, London: Routledge.

Maraspini, A.L. (1968) *The Study of an Italian Village*, Paris: Mouton.

Marnham, P. (1980) *Lourdes*, New York: Image Books.

Marvin, G. (1986) The cockfight in Andalusia, Spain, *Anthropological Quarterly* 57, 2, 60–70.

Marvin, G. (1988) *Bullfight*, Oxford: Basil Blackwell.

Mendonsa, E.L. (1982) Benefits of migration as a personal stragegy in Nazare, Portugal, *International Migration Review* 16, 3, 635–645.

Mendras, H. (1970) *The Vanishing Peasant*, Cambridge, MA: MIT Press.

Messenger, J.C. (1969) *Inis Beag*, New York: Holt, Rinehart & Winston.

Messerschmidt, D. (ed.) (1982) *Anthropologists at Home in North America*, Cambridge: Cambridge University Press.

Mewett, P. (1982a) Associated categories and the social location of relationships in a Lewis crofting community. In A.P. Cohen (ed.) *Belonging*, Manchester: Manchester University Press.

Mewett, P. (1982b) Exiles, nicknames, social identities and the production of local consciousness in a Lewis crofting comunity. In A.P. Cohen (ed.) *Belonging*, Manchester: Manchester University Press.

Miller, R.A. (1974) Are familists amoral? *American Ethnologist* 1, 515–535.

Miller, R.A. and Miller, M.G. (1978) The golden chain, *American Ethnologist* 5, 116–136.

Mingione, E. (1985) Social reproduction of the surplus labour force. In N. Redclift and E. Mingione (eds) *Beyond Employment*, Oxford: Basil Blackwell.

Moore, K. (1976a) *Those of the Street*, South Bend, IN: University of Notre Dame Press.

Moore, K. (1976b) Modernization in a Canary Island village. In J.B. Aceves and W. Douglass (eds) *The Changing Faces of Rural Spain*, New York: Wiley.

Morin, Edgar (1971) *Plodemet*, London: Allen Lane.

Moss, D. (1979) Bandits and boundaries in Sardinia, *Man* 14, 477–496.

Mulcahy, F.D. (1976) Gitano sex role symbolism and behaviour, *Anthropological Quarterly* 49, 135–151.

Murcott, A. (1982) On the social significance of the 'cooked dinner' in South Wales, *Social Science Information* 21, 677–695.

Murcott, A. (ed.) (1983) *The Sociology of Food and Eating*, Aldershot: Gower.

Murcott, A. (1988) Sociological and social anthropological approaches to food and eating, *World Review of Nutrition and Dietetics* 55, 1–40.

Murphy, M.D. (1983a) Sevillano fathers and sons, *American Ethnologist* 10, 649–664.

Murphy, M.D. (1983b) Coming of age in Seville, *Journal of Anthropological Research* 39, 4, 376–392.

Netting, R. McC. (1981) *Balancing on an Alp*, Cambridge: Cambridge University Press.

Newby, H. (1977) *The Deferential Worker*, London: Allen Lane.

O'Neill, B.J. (1983) Dying and inheriting in rural Tras-os-Montes. In P. Feijo, H. Martins and J. Pina-Cabral (eds) *Death in Portugal*, Oxford: Department of Social Anthropology.

O'Neill, B.J. (1987) *Social Inequality in a Portuguese Hamlet*, Cambridge: Cambridge University Press.

Ott, S. (1979) Aristotle among the Basques, *Man* 14, 699–711.

Ott, S. (1981) *The Circle of the Mountains*, Oxford: Clarendon Press.

Palidda, S. and Minoz, M.C. (1988) The condition of young people of foreign origin in France. In C. Wilpert (ed.) *Entering the Working World*, Aldershot: Gower.

Pardo, Italo (1989) Life, death and ambiguity in the social dynamics of inner Naples, *Man* 24, 1, 103–123.

Park, H. (1992) Passion, remembrance and identity, *Journal of Mediterranean Studies* 2, 1, 80–97.

Parman, S. (1990) *Scottish Crofters*, New York: Holt, Rinehart & Winston.

Peristiany, J.G. (1966a) Honour and shame in a Cypriot highland village. In J.G. Peristiany (ed.) *Honour and Shame*, London: Weidenfeld & Nicolson.

Peristiany, J.G. (ed.) (1966b) *Honour and Shame*, London: Weidenfeld & Nicolson.

Pina-Cabral, J. de (1986) *Sons of Adam, Daughters of Eve*, Oxford: Clarendon Press.

Pina-Cabral, J. de (1987) Paved roads and enchanted mooresses, *Man* 22, 715–733.

Pina-Cabral, J. de (1992) Against translation. In J. de Pina-Cabral and J. Campbell (eds) *Europe Observed*, London: Macmillan.

Pina-Cabral, J. de and Campbell, J. (eds) (1992) *Europe Observed*, London: Macmillan.

Pi-Sunyer, O. (1977) Changing perceptions of tourism and tourists in a Catalan coastal town. In V. Smith (ed.) *Hosts and Guests*. Philadelphia, PA: University of Pennsylvania Press.

Pi-Sunyer, O. (1978) Two stages of technological change in a Catalan fishing community. In M.E. Smith (ed.) *Those Who Live from the Sea*, St Paul, MN: West Publishing.

Pi-Sunyer, O. (1987) Town, country and nation, *Anthropological Quarterly* 60, 4, 167–173.

Pi-Sunyer, O. (1989) Changing perceptions of tourism and tourists in a Catalan resort town. In V.L. Smith (ed.) *Hosts and Guests* (2nd edition), Philadelphia, PA: University of Pennsylvania Press.

Pitkin, D.S. (1985) *The House that Giacomo Built*, Cambridge: Cambridge University Press.

Pitt-Rivers, J.A. (1954) *The People of the Sierra*, London: Weidenfeld & Nicolson (reprinted 1971 by University of Chicago Press).

Pitt-Rivers, J.A. (1976) Introduction. In J.B. Aceves and W. Douglass (eds) *The Changing Faces of Rural Spain.* New York: Wiley.

Pitt-Rivers, J.A. (1977) *The Fate of Shechem or the Politics of Sex*, Cambridge: Cambridge University Press.

Pratt, J. (1984) Christian Democrat ideology in the Cold War period. In E. Wolf (ed.) *Religion, Power and Protest*, The Hague: Mouton.

Press, I. (1979) *The City as Context*, Urbana, IL: University of Illinois Press.

Provatakis, Theoharis (n.d.) *St Dionysios of Zakynthos*, Athens: M. Toumbis.

Quastana, A.-M. and Casanova, S. (1984) Women and Corsican identity. In M. Gadant (ed.) *Women of the Mediterranean*, London: Zed.

Quintana, B. and Floyd, L. (1972) *!Que Gitano*, New York: Holt, Rinehart & Winston (reprinted 1986, Prospect Heights, IL: Waveland Press).

Rabinow, P. (1977) *Reflections on Fieldwork in Morocco*, Berkeley, CA: University of California Press.

Rapp, R. (1986) Ritual of reversion, *Critique of Anthropology* 6, 2, 35–48.

Redclift, N. and Mingione, E. (eds) (1985) *Beyond Employment*, Oxford: Basil Blackwell.

Rees, A.D. (1950) *Life in a Welsh Countryside*, Cardiff: University of Wales Press.

Rees, A. and Davies, E. (eds) (1960) *Welsh Rural Communities*, Cardiff: University of Wales Press.

Reiter, R.R. (1972) Modernization in the south of France, *Anthropological Quarterly* 45, 35–43.

Rex, J., Joly, D. and Wilpert, C. (eds) (1988) *Immigrant Associations in Europe*, Aldershot: Gower.

Rhoades, R.E. (1978) Intra-European return migration and rural development, *Human Organization* 37, 2, 136–147.

Rhoades, R.E. (1979a) From caves to main street. In R.E. Rhoades (ed.) *The Anthropology of Return Migration.* Special Issue of *Papers in Anthropology* 20, 1.

Rhoades, R.E. (ed.) (1979b) *The Anthropology of Return Migration.* Special Issue of *Papers in Anthropology* 20, 1.

Riegelhaupt, J.F. (1967) Saloio women, *Anthropological Quarterly* 40, 109–126.

Riegelhaupt, J. (1984) Popular anticlericalism and religiosity. In E. Wolf (ed.) *Religion, Power and Protest in Local Communities*, Berlin: Mouton.

Roden, C. (1970) *A Book of Middle Eastern Food*, Harmondsworth: Penguin.

Rogers, S.C. (1975) Female forms of power and the myth of male dominance, *American Ethnologist* 1, 4, 727–756.

Rogers, S.C. (1985) Gender in southwestern France. In D. Gilmore and G. Gwynne (eds) *Sex and Gender in Southern Europe*, A Special Issue of *Anthropology* 9, 1 and 2, 68–86.

Rogers, S.C. (1987) Good to think *Anthropological Quarterly* 60, 2, 56–63.

Rogers, S.C. (1991) *Shaping Modern Times in Rural France*, Princeton, NJ: Princeton University Press.

Romanucci-Ross, Lola (1991) *One Hundred Towers*, London: Bergin & Garvey.

Rosen, H. and Burgess, T. (1980) *Languages and Dialects of London School Children*. London: Ward Lock.

Rosenberg, H. (1988) *A Negotiated World*, Toronto: Toronto University Press.

Rosenberg, H., Reiter, R.B. and Reiter, R.R. (1973) Peasants working in French Alpine tourism, *Studies in European Society* 1, 21–38.

Sachs, L. (1983) *Evil eye and bacteria: Turkish migrant women and Swedish health care*. Stockholm: University of Stockholm Department of Social Anthropology.

Salamone, S.D. (1986) *In the Shadow of the Holy Mountain*, Boulder, CO: East European Monographs.

Sanchis, P. (1983) The Portuguese *romarias*. In S. Wilson (ed.) *Saints and their Cults*, Cambridge: Cambridge University Press.

Sanmartin, R. (1982) Marriage and inheritance in a Mediterranean fishing community, *Man* 17, 664–72.

Scheper-Hughes, N. (1979) *Saints, Scholars and Schizophrenics*, Berkeley: University of California Press.

Schmitt, Jean-Claude (1983) *The Holy Greyhound*, Cambridge: Cambridge University Press.

Schneider, J. (1971) Of vigilance and virgins, *Ethnology* 9, 1–24.

Schneider, J. and Schneider, P. (1976) *Culture and Political Economy in Western Sicily*, New York: Academic Press.

Schweizer, Peter (1988) *Shepherds, Workers, Intellectuals: Culture and Centre–Periphery Relationship in a Sardinian Village*. Stockholm: University of Stockholm Dept. of Anthropology.

Segalen, Martine (1983) *Love and Power in the Peasant Family*, Oxford: Basil Blackwell.

Segalen, Martine (1991) *Fifteen generations of Bretons*, Cambridge: Cambridge University Press.

Seremetakis, C. Nadia (1991) *The Last Word*, Chicago: University of Chicago Press.

Sheehan, E.A. (1993) The student of culture and the ethnography of Irish intellectuals. In C.B. Brettell (ed.) *When They Read What We Write*, London: Bergin & Garvey.

Silverman, S. (1968) Agricultural organization, social structure and values in Italy, *American Anthropologist* 70, 1–20.

Silverman, S. (1975) *Three Bells of Civilisation*, New York: Columbia University Press.

Silverman, S. (1977) Patronage as myth. In E. Gellner and J. Waterbury (eds) *Patrons and Clients in Mediterranean Societies*, London: Duckworth.

Simic, A. (1983) Urbanization and modernization in Yugoslavia. In M. Kenny and D. Kertzer (eds) *Urban Life in Mediterranean Europe*, Urbana, IL: University of Illinois Press.

Simon, K.E. (1976) *Outmigration, Depopulation and Social Change in Rural Corsica*, Ann Arbor, MI: UMI.

Slater, Candace (1986) *Trail of Miracles*, Berkeley, CA: University of California Press.

Slater, Candace (1990) *City Steeple, City Streets*, Berkeley: University of California Press.

Smith, V.L. (ed.) (1989) *Hosts and Guests*, (2nd edition) Philadelphia: University of Pennsylvania Press.

Sontz, A.H.L. (1987) Factory and community in a West German immigrant neighbourhood. In H.C. Buechler and J.M. Buechler (eds) *Migrants in Europe*, New York: Greenwood Press.

Spangler, M. (1983) Urban research in Yugoslavia. In M. Kenny and D. Kertzer (eds) *Urban Life in Mediterranean Europe*, Urbana, IL: University of Illinois Press.

Spindler, G. (1973) *Burgbach*, New York: Holt, Rinehart & Winston.

Spindler, G. and Spindler, L. (eds) (1987) Schonhausen revisted and the rediscovery of culture. In G. and L. Spindler (eds) *Interpretive Ethnography of Education*, London: Erlbaum.

Stewart, Charles (1991) *Demons and the Devil*, Princeton, NJ: Princeton University Press.

Strathern, M. (1981) *Kinship at the Core*, Cambridge: Cambridge University Press.

Sutton, S.B. (1983) Rural–urban migration in Greece. In M. Kenny and D. Kertzer (eds) *Urban Life in Mediterranean Europe*, Urbana, IL: University of Illinois Press.

Tannen, D. (1991) *You Just Don't Understand*, London: Virago.

Tapper, N. (1990) 'Ziyaret'. In D.F. Eickelman and J. Piscatori (eds) *Muslim Travellers*, London: Routledge.

Tentori, T. (1976) Social classes and family in a Southern Italian town: Matera. In J.G. Peristiany (ed.) *Mediterranean Family Structures*, Cambridge: Cambridge University Press.

Thomas, Beth (1987) Accounting for language shift in a South Wales mining community, *Cardiff Working Papers in Welsh Linguistics No. 5*, 55–99.

Thomas, Peter Wynne (1986) The impact of S4C on Welsh-speaking schoolchildren. Proceedings of the Conference on 'Lesser-used Languages and Information Media in the European Community: Problems of Radio and Television', held in Sardinia, October. Published by ISPROM, Brussels, pp. 317–326.

Thomas, Peter Wynne (1987) S4C – Sianel Plant Cymru? *Cardiff Working Papers in Welsh Linguistics No. 5*, 101–128.

Thornton, Mary A. (1987) *Sekt* versus *Schnapps* in an Austrian village. In M. Douglas (ed.) *Constructive Drinking*, Cambridge: Cambridge University Press.

Thubron, C. (1986) *Journey into Cyprus*, Harmondsworth: Penguin.

Thuren, B.M. (1988) *Left Hand Left Behind*, Stockholm: University of Stockholm Department of Anthropology.

Tunstall, J. (1972) *The Fisherman* (3rd edition), London: MacGibbon & Kee.

Turner, V. and Turner, E. (1978) *Image and Pilgrimage in Christian Culture*, New York: Columbia University Press.

Turney-High, H.H. (1953) *Chateau-Gerard*, Columbia, SC: University of South Carolina Press.

Uhl, S.C. (1985) Special friends. In D. Gilmore and G. Gwynne (eds) *Sex and Gender in Southern Europe.* A Special Issue of *Anthropology* 9, 1 and 2, 129–152.

Urla, J. (1987) *Being Basque, Speaking Basque,* Ann Arbor, MI: UMI.

Van Gennep, A. (1908) *The Rites of Passage* (English translation, 1960), London: Routledge.

van Ginkel, Rob (1989) Plunderers into planters. In J. Boissevain and J. Verrips (eds) *Dutch Dilemmas,* Maastricht: Van Gorcum.

van Ginkel, Rob (1991) The Sea of Bitterness, *Man* 26, 4, 691–707.

Vermuelen, H. (1983) Urban research in Greece. In M. Kenny and D. Kertzer (eds) *Urban Life in Mediterranean Europe,* Urbana, IL: University of Illinois Press.

Verrips, J. (1975) The decline of small-scale farming in a Dutch village. In J. Boissevain and E. Friedl (eds) *Beyond the Community,* The Hague: Mouton.

Victor, J.S. (1993) *Satanic Panic: The Creation of a Contemporary Legend.* Chicago, IL: Open Court.

Villepontoux, E.J. (1981) *Tourism and Social Change in a French Alpine Community,* London: UMI.

Wade, R. (1971) Political behaviour and world view in a central Italian village. In F.G. Bailey (ed.) *Gifts and Poison,* Oxford: Basil Blackwell.

Waterbury, J. (1972) *North for the Trade,* Berkeley, CA: University of California Press.

Watson, J. (ed.) (1977) *Between Two Cultures.* Oxford: Basil Blackwell.

Weinberg, D. (1975) *Peasant Wisdom,* Berkeley, CA: University of California Press.

Weingrod, A. (1968) Patrons, patronage, and political parties, *Comparative Studies in Society and History* 10, 376–400.

White, C. (1980) *Patrons and Partisans,* Cambridge: Cambridge University Press.

Whitehead, A. (1976) Sexual antagonism in Herefordshire. In D.L. Barker and S. Allen (eds) *Dependence and Exploitation in Work and Marriage,* London: Tavistock.

Williams, G. and Thomas, A.R. (1985) *A Report of Research into the Effects of S4C on the Welsh Language,* Bangor, University College of North Wales for the Welsh Education Office.

Williams, Tim (1987) Futile linguistic engineering, *Times Educational Supplement,* 20 February: 20.

Williams, W.M. (1956) *The Sociology of an English Village,* London: Routledge.

Wilpert, C. (ed.) (1988a) *Entering the Working World,* Aldershot: Gower.

Wilpert, C. (1988b) Work and the second generation. In C. Wilpert (ed.) *Entering the Working World,* Aldershot: Gower.

Wilson, S. (ed.) (1983a) *Saints and their Cults,* Cambridge: Cambridge University Press.

Wilson, S. (1983b) Cults of the saints in the churches of central Paris. In S. Wilson (ed.) *Saints and their Cults,* Cambridge: Cambridge University Press.

Wise, M. (1984) *The Common Fisheries Policy of the European Community,* London: Methuen.

Woolard, K.A. (1988) Language variation and cultural hegemony, *American Ethnologist* 12,4, 738–748.

Woolard, K.A. (1989) *Double Talk*, Stanford: Stanford University Press.

Wylie, L. (1957) *Village in the Vancluse*, Cambridge, MA: Harvard University Press (3rd edition 1975).

Wylie, L. (ed.) (1966) *Chanzeaux*, Ann Arbor, MI: UMI.

Young, M. and Wilmott, P. (1957) *Family and Kinship in East London*, London: Routledge.

Yucel, A.E. (1987) Turkish migrant workers in the Federal Republic of Germany. In H.C. Buechler and J.M. Buechler (eds) *Migrants in Europe*, New York: Greenwood Press.

Zinovieff, Sophie (1991a) Inside out and outside in, *Journal of Mediterranean Studies* 1, 1, 120–134.

Zinovieff, Sophie (1991b) Hunters and hunted. In P. Loizos and E. Papataxiarchis (eds) *Contested Identities*, Princeton, NJ: Princeton University Press.

Zonabend, F. (1984) *The Enduring Memory*, Manchester: Manchester University Press.

Zonabend, F. (1993) *The Nuclear Peninsula*, Cambridge: Cambridge University Press.

Name index

Subject index